CHAKRAS:
WHAT THEY REALLY ARE

A Brief and Concrete Explanation with the Help of Science, Tantra Yoga and Modern Psychology Insights

Stéphane Le Colas

Copyright © 2018 Stéphane Le Colas

All rights reserved.

ISBN: 9781980659181

TABLE OF CONTENTS

CHAKRAS: WHAT THEY REALLY ARE

1 INTRODUCTION

As a yoga teacher, Yoga therapist and Ayurvedic practitioner, I often hear many things about the Chakras from my students or from my patients. It happens that there is a lot of misinformation out there.

I conceived this book as a training course on Yogic Cosmology and Chakras and I assume you already have some basis in Yoga.

I have compiled much information, both from Westerners and Easterners, coming from different cultures and traditions.

With the main understandings of the Yogic Cosmologies, from the history of the Chakras, to their meanings, passing through their « treatment », I really hope you will find in this book the information you are looking for.

As the 2nd Chakra is involved in 2 big curses of our modern days – trauma and addiction – a special emphasis is put on them.

I also hope that you will then peacefully spread the word: « No, the 1st Chakra is not red... »

2 YOGIC COSMOLOGY
THE MANIFESTATION AND EVOLUTION OF CONSCIOUSNESS

Before going straight to the Chakras, we have to explain a bit about yogic cosmology for a better understanding.
Cosmology is the study of the universe in its totality and by extension, humanity's place in it. Though the word cosmology is recent, the study of the universe has a long history involving science, philosophy, esotericism and religion.

Cosmology can help us answer questions like:
- What is the world?
- How does it come into existence?
- How does the world function?
- What is the purpose of human existence?

Within the wide field of yoga philosophy, there are different versions of cosmology. These differ not only in terms of details, but also in terms of what they offer as the meaning of the universe.
We will briefly study here 2 of the most famous cosmologies, Samkhya and Kashmiri Shaivist Cosmology. These cosmologies are

said to have been perceived by yogis who were able to expand their minds out into the corners of the universe and thereby understand the mechanisms of life. We are looking at this based on our inference that their authority is accurate.

For various personal, social and cultural reasons some seers have been able to perceive certain aspects and have interpreted them accordingly. Hence, we find discrepancies between different cosmologies.

I/ SAMKHYA COSMOLOGY

Samkya is the first real school of philosophy in India. Founded by Kapil. It influenced both Buddhism and Classical Yoga. In Samkhya, we do not find no mention of a divine source, every entity is an eternal Purusa in and of itself. This posits that people lack discriminative knowledge – but it is the key to the truth of our eternal nature. Samkhya is a fundamentally dualistic philosophy (Dvaita rather than Advaita) and duality is expressed through: Purusa (unqualified) and Prakritti (with qualities).

In this cosmology, the Gunas are the 3 qualities of everything in the expressed universe. These 3 qualities are:
- Sattva, which is sentient, alive, fresh, alert and subtle. For example, an Awakened person is said to be pure Sattvic.
- Rajas, which is dynamic, active and mutative. For example, the Animal kingdom is said to be Rajasic.
- Tamas, which is static, dull, lazy and exhausted. For example, the Mineral kingdom is said to be Tamasic.

In Nature, the Gunas exist in everything in different proportion. Neither one is good or bad. However, as a Human, we should be looking to be more and more Sattvic.

Beside these qualities, everything expressed in the universe is made of various components, the Tattvas. The number and definition of the Tattvas differ depending on which school of thought you are looking at. They are used to explain both Samkhya (24 Tattvas) and Kashmiri Shaivism (36 Tattvas) cosmologies.

However, both recognised the 5 Great Elements, the Mahatattvas, as the final points of manifestation. These 5 gross elements are:
- Akasha, Ether/Space, the Ethereal factor.
- Vayu, Air, the Aerial factor.
- Tejas, Fire, the Luminous factor.
- Apa, Water, the Liquid factor.
- Ksiti, Earth, the Solid factor.

The principle of causality is a key point in understanding the Samkhya philosophy. It comes from the idea that nothing can really be created from or destroyed into nothingness. There is no concept of a creator or God (later, in the Yoga Sutras, Patanjali propounds the idea of an impersonal Supreme, Parama Purusa). Their liberation (Moksa) occurs through discriminative knowledge – which is basically a true understanding of the Tattvas.

At the top of the Samkhya cosmology, we have Purusa (unqualified, pure consciousness) and Prakritti (the operative principle). Prakritti unfolds through the 24 Tattvas « in order to please » Purusa.

Actually, we can draft the cosmology in this way:

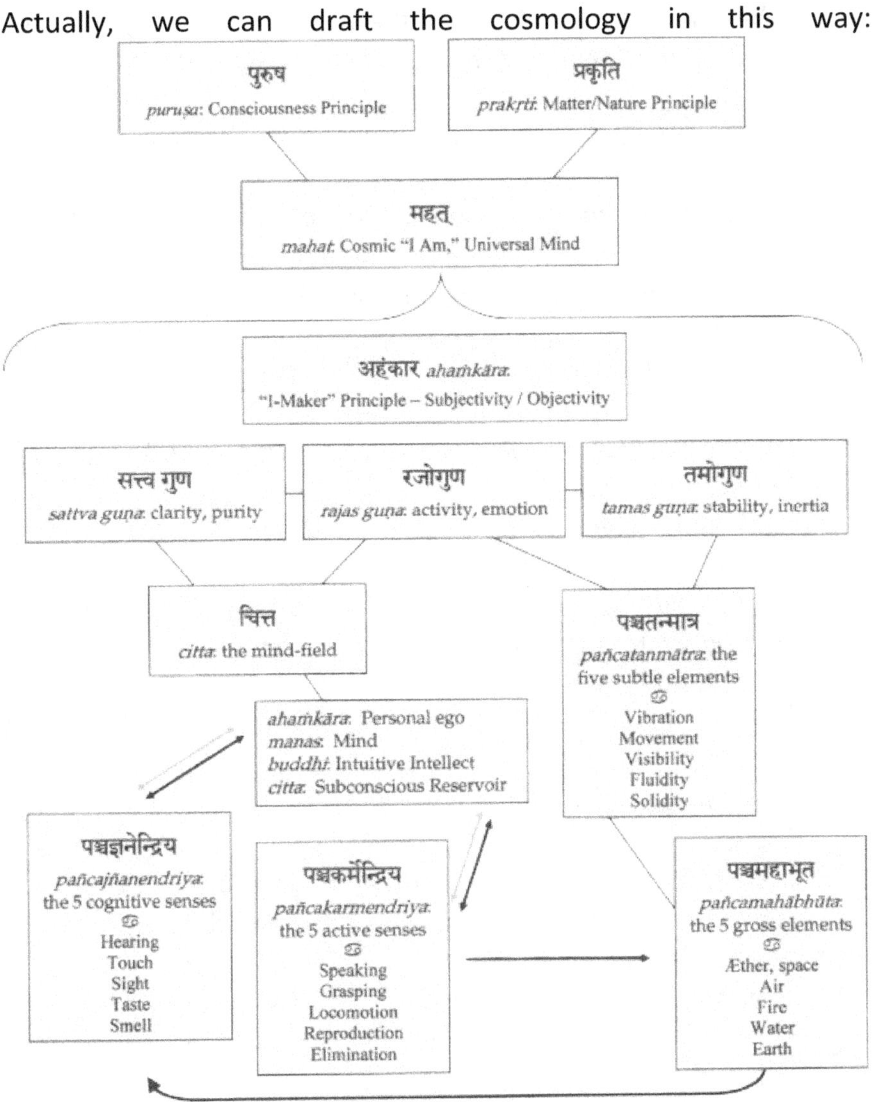

Prakritti is the first element. It is the most subtle potentiality that is the source of whatever exists in the physical universe.

Mind unfolds out of Prakriti into:

- Mahat: Higher mind
- then Ahamkara: Ego or "I"-ness

Out of the Ahamkara and through the Gunas, the other elements evolve, including Manas: the mind, and Buddhi which is intuition, 6th sense.

The 5 sense organs (Pancha Jnana Indriya) then unfold from the sattvic aspect of Ahamkara (ego). They are:

1. Hearing, which echoes in the Ethereal Factor and in the 5th Chakra.
2. Feeling, which echoes in the Aerial Factor and in the 4th Chakra.
3. Seeing, which echoes in the Luminous Factor and in the 3rd Chakra.
4. Tasting, which echoes in the Liquid Factor and in the 2nd Chakra.
5. Smelling, which echoes in the Solid Factor and in the 1st Chakra.

The 5 motor organs (Pancha Karma Indriya) also unfold from the sattvic aspect of the ego (Ahamkara). They are:

1. Arms and hands
2. Legs and feet
3. Vocal chords
4. Urino-genital organs
5. Anus

From the static (Tamasic) aspect of ego (Ahamkara) unfold the 5 subtle elements (Pancha Tanmatras). These subtle elements are the root energies of:

1. Sound
2. Touch
3. Sight
4. Taste
5. Smell

Regarding Yoga, Patanjali who was the first to really define it, drew from Samkhya to write the Yoga Sutras. He says that Yoga is the corralling of the modifications of the mind (Yogash Citta Vrtti Nirodah, Y.S.1.2).

Yoga is thus the achievement of folding the Tattvas back up in order to abide in the eternal, immutable nature of Purusa.

II/ KASHMIRI SHAIVIST COSMOLOGY

Kashmiri Shaivism emerged around 700 C.E. from ancient Shaivist teachings but it renewed interest in the past 100 years. It is a part of the more general Shaivist religion/path, which is the oldest spiritual path in India.

The Kashmiri Shaivism cosmology is a Tantric one with a different beginning of creation. It starts with Paramashiva (Brahman), the unmanifested Consciousness, then Shiva (the Cognitive Principle) and Shakti (the Operative Principle), the manifest godheads.
The important distinction between Samkhya and Kashmiri Shaivism is the inclusion, before Purusa and Prakritti of a multifaceted cosmic mind.

I will not describe here all the cosmology but you can have a general overview of it on the following diagrams:

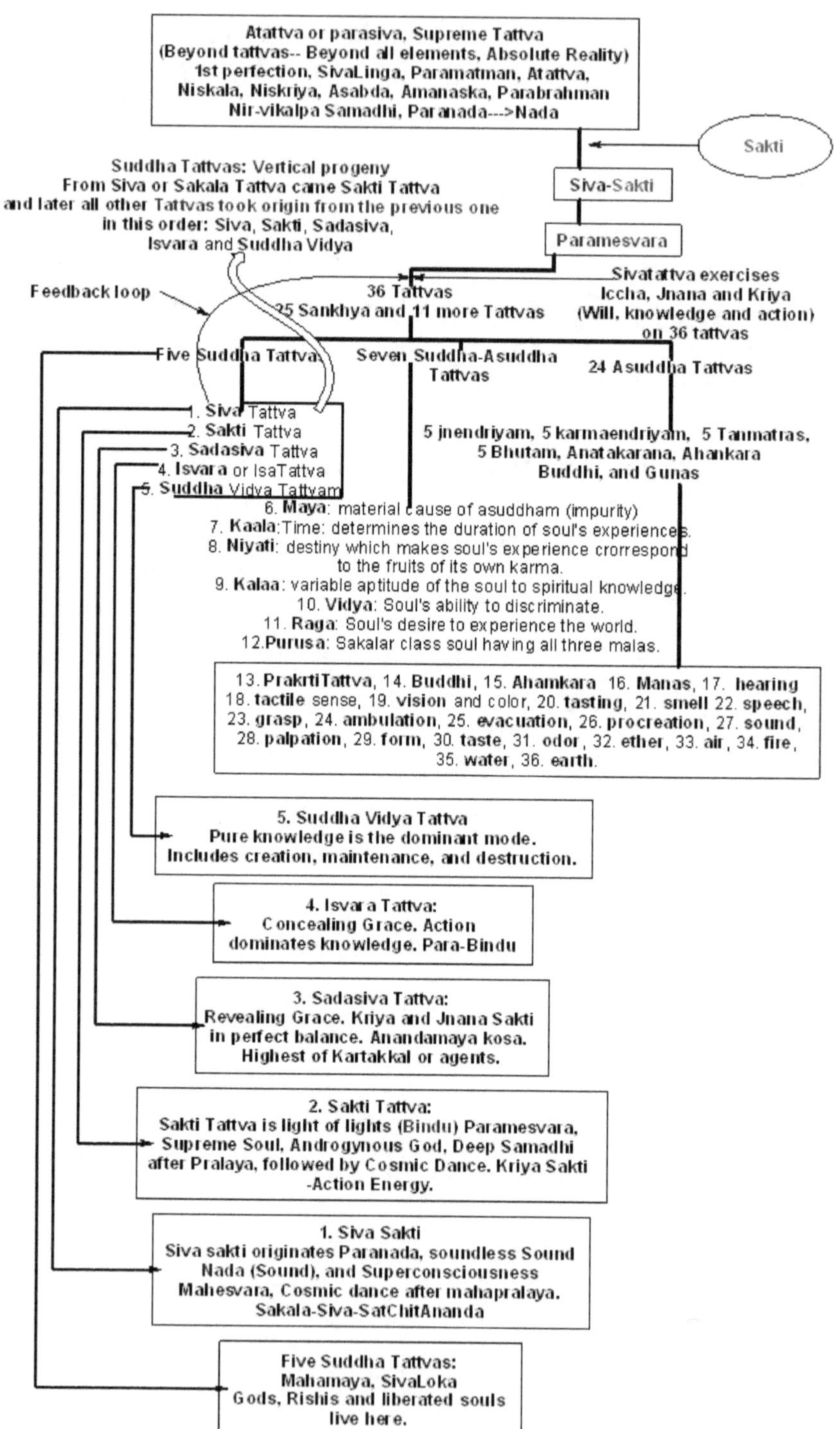

Atattva or parasiva, Supreme Tattva
(Beyond tattvas-- Beyond all elements, Absolute Reality)
1st perfection, SivaLinga, Paramatman, Atattva,
Niskala, Niskriya, Asabda, Amanaska, Parabrahman
Nir-vikalpa Samadhi, Paranada--->Nada
Sakti
Siva-Sakti
Paramesvara
Suddha Tattvas: Vertical progeny
From Siva or Sakala Tattva came Sakti Tattva
and later all other Tattvas took origin from the previous one
in this order: Siva, Sakti, Sadasiva,
Isvara and Suddha Vidya
Feedback loop
36 Tattvas
35 Sankhya and 11 more Tattvas
Sivatattva exercises
Iccha, Jnana and Kriya
(Will, knowledge and action)
on 36 tattvas
Five Suddha Tattva
Seven Suddha-Asuddha Tattvas
24 Asuddha Tattvas
1. Siva Tattva
2. Sakti Tattva
3. Sadasiva Tattva
4. Isvara or IsaTattva
5. Suddha Vidya Tattvam
5 jnendriyam, 5 karmaendriyam, 5 Tanmatras,
5 Bhutam, Anatakarana, Ahankara
Buddhi, and Gunas
6. Maya: material cause of asuddham (impurity)
7. Kaala:Time: determines the duration of soul's experiences.
8. Niyati: destiny which makes soul's experience crorrespond
to the fruits of its own karma.
9. Kalaa: variable aptitude of the soul to spiritual knowledge.
10. Vidya: Soul's ability to discriminate.
11. Raga: Soul's desire to experience the world.
12.Purusa: Sakalar class soul having all three malas.
13. PrakrtiTattva, 14. Buddhi, 15. Ahamkara 16. Manas, 17. hearing
18. tactile sense, 19. vision and color, 20. tasting, 21. smell 22. speech,
23. grasp, 24. ambulation, 25. evacuation, 26. procreation, 27. sound,
28. palpation, 29. form, 30. taste, 31. odor, 32. ether, 33. air, 34. fire,
35. water, 36. earth.
5. Suddha Vidya Tattva
Pure knowledge is the dominant mode.
Includes creation, maintenance, and destruction.
4. Isvara Tattva:
Concealing Grace. Action
dominates knowledge. Para-Bindu
3. Sadasiva Tattva:
Revealing Grace. Kriya and Jnana Sakti
in perfect balance. Anandamaya kosa.
Highest of Kartakkal or agents.
2. Sakti Tattva:
Sakti Tattva is light of lights (Bindu) Paramesvara,
Supreme Soul, Androgynous God. Deep Samadhi
after Pralaya, followed by Cosmic Dance. Kriya Sakti
-Action Energy.
1. Siva Sakti
Siva sakti originates Paranada, soundless Sound
Nada (Sound), and Superconsciousness
Mahesvara, Cosmic dance after mahapralaya.
Sakala-Siva-SatChitAnanda
Five Suddha Tattvas:
Mahamaya, SivaLoka
Gods, Rishis and liberated souls
live here.

CHAKRAS: WHAT THEY REALLY ARE

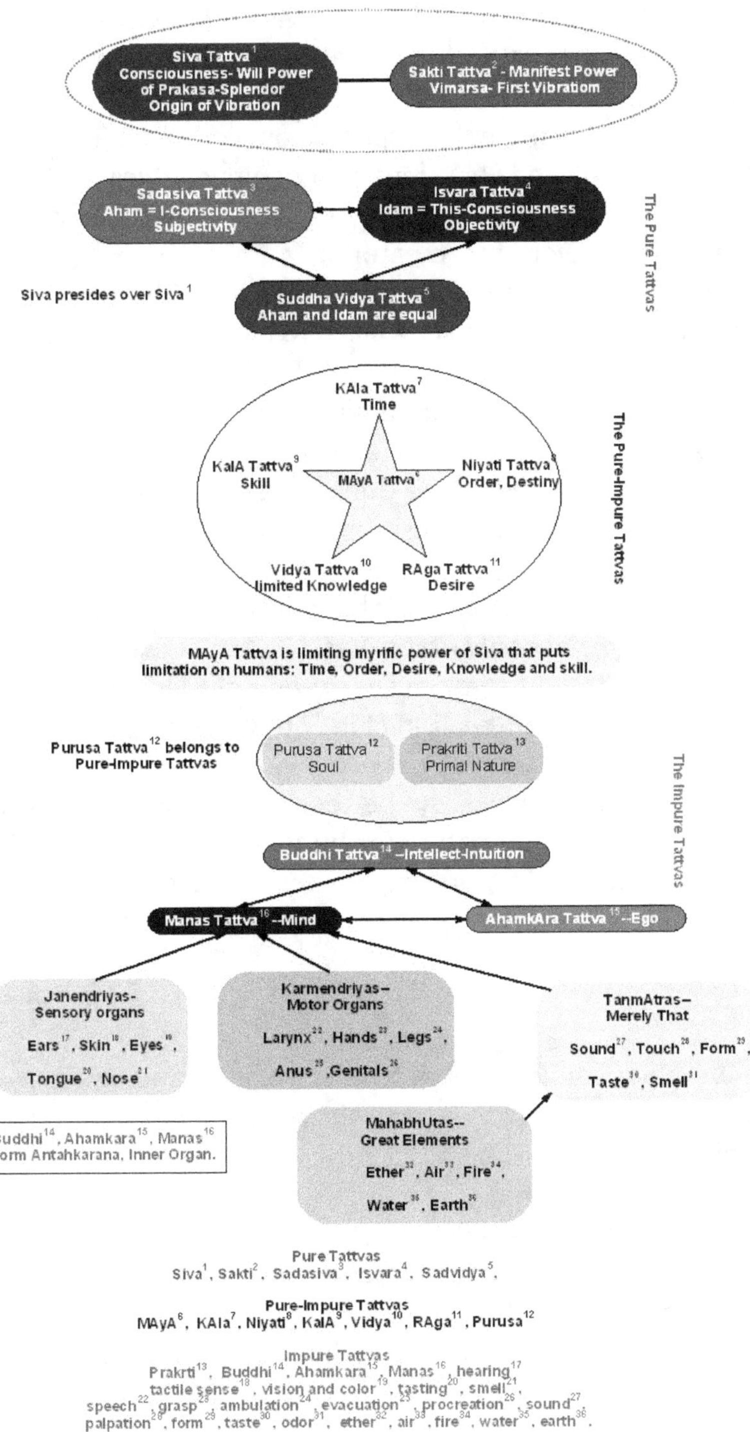

The other important distinctions between the 2 cosmologies to understand are that, in Kashmiri Shaivism:

- The Cosmic Mind is composed of:

1) Sadashiva, "I am this" (emphasis on I, the subjective. Sada means "Truth" and Shiva means "Cognitive Principle".)
2) Ishvara, "This I am" (emphasis is on "This" the objective. Ishvara is the word for "creator".)
3) Suddhavidya, "True knowledge" (the state of balance between the subject and the object which are now clearly distinct in the one.)

- Out of Suddhavidya emerges Maya (illusion), which is the beginning of dualism. Prakritti is the first stage of Maya and is controlled by the Gunas – Sattva, Rajas and Tamas.

The rest of the Kashmiri Shaivism system follows Samkhya.

According to Kashmiri Shaivism, the individual must realize that it is Pure consciousness only that exists.

Like Samkhya it is unconsciousness, or delusion by maya, that keeps the aspirant from realizing his or her true nature.

According to Tantra, which can be seen as the Kashmiri Shaivism's integral way of transformation for human beings, the meaning of life is to be found in pursuing balance between living in this expressed universe while we attempt to understand who we truly are.

Once we have studied the two main Yogic cosmologies, we can deduct from them some practical applications and concluding principles.

- Universe of Desire: It is the desire of the Divine to express itself as the material world. It is the desire of every entity to merge with the Supreme.

  All desires are veiled expressions of this one desire.

- Matter and Life: Life has evolved out of matter because matter has evolved out of Cosmic Mind.
- Evolution from the last 2 points:
  1. Prakriti (through the medium of prana) causes the 5 factors to organize themselves into more and more complex forms of life.
  2. Mind begins to evolve out of matter. It was always there, just dormant.
  3. Consciousness evolves out of mind.
- Pressure:
  1. It is the pressure of the Tamasic Prakritti acting on the fundamental factors that makes life happen.
  2. Likewise, it is periods of pressure that cause growth. That is the case with the pressure from the amniotic fluid which causes a baby to develop. That is also why massage/touch is essential to infants/children for proper growth and development.
  3. Pressure comes in a variety of forms. For humans pressure is physical, psychic and spiritual. When stressed we say, "I'm under a lot of pressure."
  4. Pressure is responsible for evolution. In other words, life's obstacles are our friends.
  This is a quintessentially tantric view of life.
- Evolution from Pressure:
  1. Life becomes increasingly more complex under pressure from Cosmic Mind.
  2. It's the desire of Mind to create more and more complex structures which can house the evolving mind. The physical structure evolves because of this desire.
- Evolution of Mind:
  1. Mind begins to evolve out of matter. (It has been latent within it).
  2. Consciousness will evolve out of mind.
- Instinct:

1. Less developed beings evolve due to physical pressure in the world. They are controlled by a more unconscious part of the mind.

2. There is a stronger sense of the object than of the self. This leads to instinctual action or reaction.

3. The desire is self-preservation, self-reproduction.

- Intellect:

  1. The Ego emerges. More developed beings have a sense of ego, or "I-ness."

  2. The structure is more complex and has a more developed neuro-endocrine system to deal with the complexity of thought.

  3. More developed beings evolve through the pressure of intellect.

- Intuition:

  1. The witness emerges from the ego due to the influence of the Sattva Guna (it was always there, just latent).

  The feeling of "I am" develops. The being is more intuitional, contemplative.

  2. The being evolves due to internal spiritual pressure/desire.

- The Thirst for Limitlessness:

  1. In the being in which the witness dominates, the mind begins to develop a strong desire for the infinite.

  2. The mind literally expands.There is a change in mass and volume of the mental body.

  3. The physical structure also changes — a more complex neuro-endocrine system is necessary to accommodate the increasing desire for expansion.

- Subtlety increases: If we spend all our time in the part of us that associates with what we have done (the ego) we cannot develop the witness. We are externally focused.

- Samadhi:

1. When the whole of the mind is eventually converted into the witness this is called Savikalpa Samadhi (qualified Oneness).

2. When the witness is converted into the Soul (Atman), it is now beyond the binding force of the 3 qualities (Gunas) and this is called Nirvikalpa Samadhi (unqualified Oneness). This state is beyond the mind.

This understanding of the different steps of Tantra and Kashmiri Shaivism is essential to approach the meanings and functions of the Chakras.

3 WHAT ARE THE CHAKRAS?

Chakra is the Sanskrit word for « wheel ». They are then physical-psychological-spiritual wheels or vortices.

The word is pronounced « Tchak.Ra » or « \ ˈchä-krə » in phonetic.

We can find different definitions of the Chakras, depending of the original tradition which is talking about them.

Harish Johari, who was an eminent Indian tantric specialist of the Chakras and author of many books related to them says that they are « centers for transforming mental/emotional energy into spiritual energy ».

Sir Jon Woodroffe (Arthur Avalon), who was an English indianist, wrote in his book *The Serpent Power* that the Chakras are « powers of the various *Tattvas* or Principles ».

Indeed, we can say that they are an interface between mind, body and spirit.
They are related to physical structures where consciousness "plugs into" the body. Actually, Chakras can manifest through neuroendocrine activity.

They create every system in the body. They are the holographic, energetic blueprint of the physical body, as well as the mind and spirit.

From a yogic point of view, Chakras communicate via the nadis, which are subtle energetic pathways. Nadis run through connective tissue (fascia). This communication may be scientifically explained through PNI (psychoneuroimmunology).
Yogis understood that Chakras are related to mental/emotional states and that when they are not functioning properly, the mind is imbalanced.

It seems important here to come back to what Sir Jon Woodroffe wrote: Chakras would be the way in which the 5 elements organize themselves in living beings to create life with the help of prana.

As a reminder, the 5 Greats Elements are :
- Space   Ethereal (*Akasha*)
- Air   Aerial (*Vayu*)
- Fire   Luminous (*Tejas*)
- Water   Liquid (*Api*)
- Earth   Solid (*Ksiti*)

4 CHAKRAS AND THE TANTRICS

Many of the first scriptures we have on the Chakras come from the Tantra philosophy.

Regarding Tantra, the cosmic elements vibrate universally – vibrations create specific shapes, colors, and sounds. Thus, the key to balancing the Chakras is to bring them into harmony with the cosmic vibrations of the universal elements.

The Tantrics described many colors in each Chakra, but they considered the color of the element (the tattva) the most helpful in balancing the Chakra.

When your elements vibrate in harmony with the universe, your Chakras are balanced. This is the practice of Tantra. For the tantric yogi, attending to Chakra imbalance is the work of life.

The name of each Chakra is a Sanskrit word. Here are their names, from bottom to top, and their English translation:

1st Chakra	Muladhara	The Root Support
2nd Chakra	Svadhisthana	One's Own Abode
3rd Chakra	Manipura	The Jeweled City
4th Chakra	Anahata	The Unstruck
5th Chakra	Vishuddha	The Pure Center

6th Chakra   Ajna   The Command Center
7th Chakra   Sahasrara   The Thousand-Petaled Lotus

Still according to Tantra, each Chakra have archetypes composed of gods, goddesses and animals which are representations of energies associated with each Chakra.
The archetypes are vehicles to understanding the essence of the Chakra.

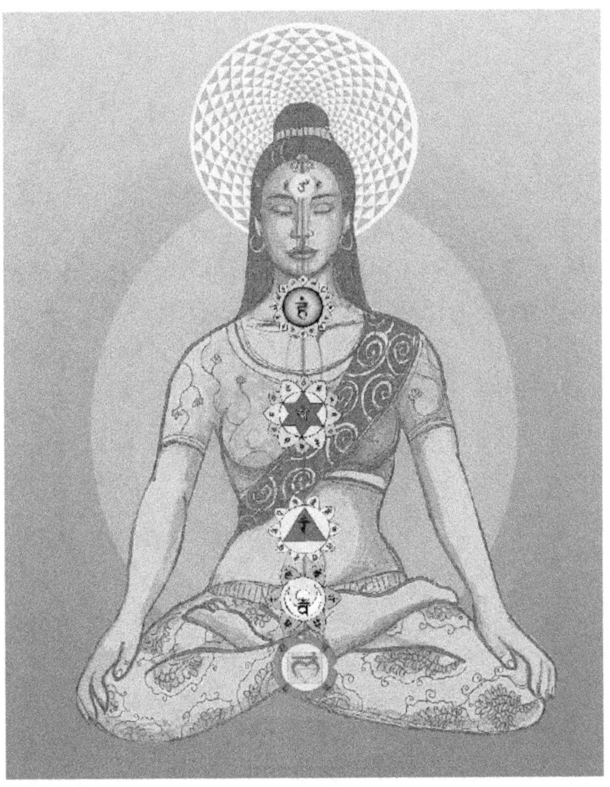

5 HISTORY OF THE CHAKRAS

In early Buddhist and Shaivist Tantra (around 200 c.e.) there is a concept of four Chakras located in the lower region, at the navel level, at the heart level, and at the head level.

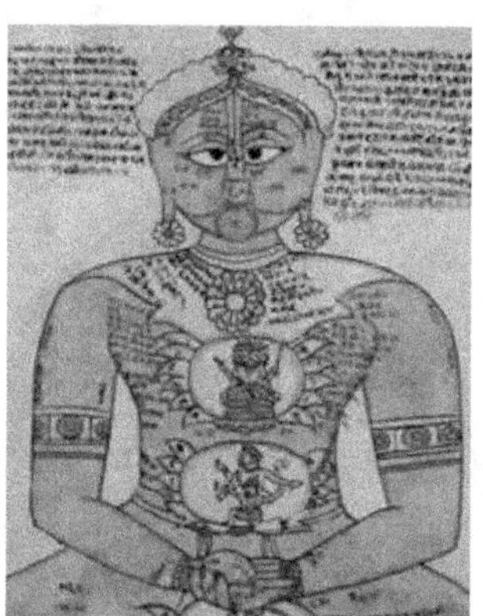

We also find notions of Chakras in Egypt. Joseph Campbell, who was an American author and professor in mythology, explains the Ancient Egyptian's understanding of the Chakras - the animals rules the lower three. (Mythos II) The Ancient Mayan culture had some understanding of the Chakra system too. Yok'hah in Yucatec Maya, means yok' (above or on top of) and hah (truth), very similar to the Sanskrit word *yoga* ("yoked" to Oneness)...

However, the system of the 7 Chakras we know today seems to have been developed in the early period of the Natha cult (perhaps 1200 c.e.). The Nathas were the first to develop yoga practices to purify the Chakras.

> *"When all the nadis and Chakras*
> *which are full of impurities are*
> *purified, then the yogis is able to*
> *retain prana."*
> (Hatha Yoga Pradipika 2.5)

The two first real works on the Chakras were composed in the 16th century with information from the 6th to 15th centuries. They are the *Sat Cakra Nirupama* ("The Description of the Six Centers") and the *Padaka Pancaka* ("The Five-fold Footstool").

The Serpent Power, published in 1919, is the book which introduced the Chakras to the Western world.

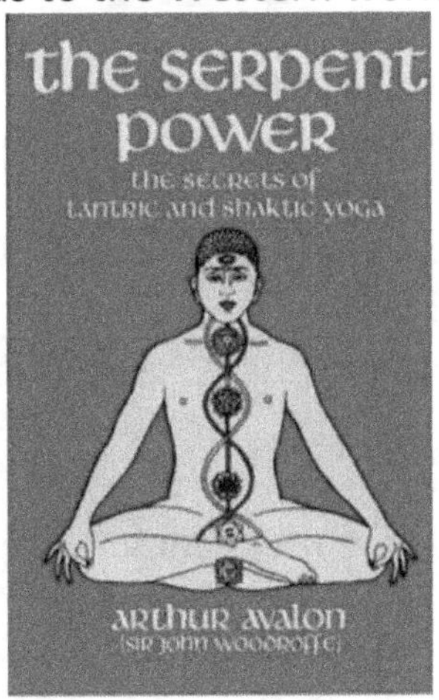

In 1927, Charles Leadbeater, an early Theosophist, wrote *The Chakras*. Leadbeater was the first to suggest that Chakras are able to be "seen" by others, through clairvoyance. He also moved the position of the third and fourth Chakras.

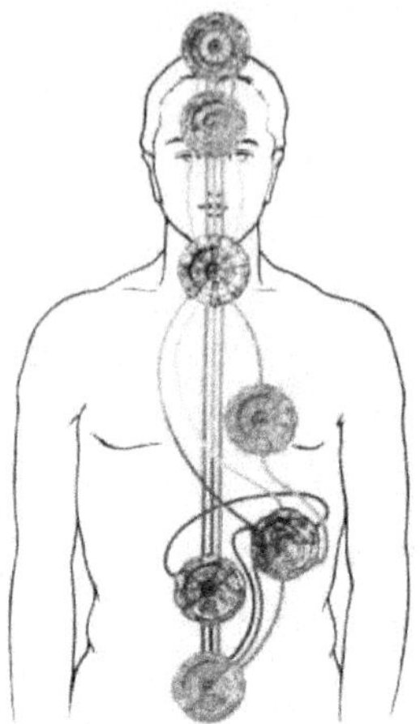

Leadbeater's work sets the stage for a New Age Chakra perspective: We can heal other's Chakras through energy and intuitive work.
Prior to this, yogic Chakra work was only done through intuitive practice on yourself (or through the work of a realized being).

Then, it was the famous psychologist Carl Gustav Jung who talked about the Chakras during 4 lectures he gave in Zurich in 1932. Jung interpreted the Indian metaphors for a Western audience. He defined his work as the integration of Eastern thought with Western psycho-analytical principles.
However, Jung's work on the Chakras remained obscure for decades.

Working somehow in the path of Jung, Joseph Campbell offered a fascinating interpretation of the images in the Chakra system.
Indeed, archetypes of the Chakras are composed of male and female deities, shapes, sounds objects and animals which are representations of energies associated with each Chakra.
These symbols are vehicles which transport the yogi to the essence of the Chakra.

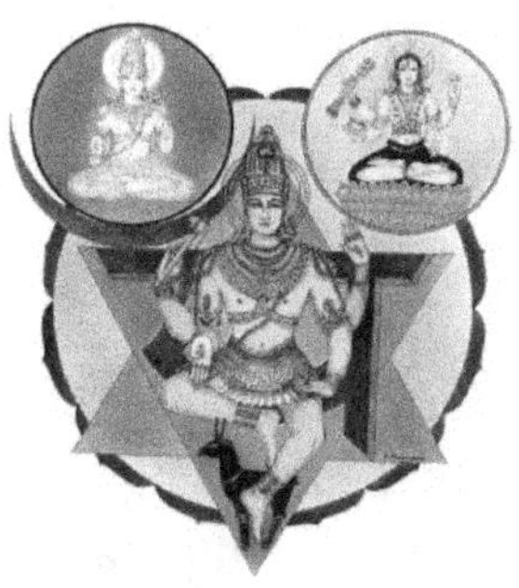

In the 1970's, Rajneesh (later known as Osho), a trained psychologist, made the idea that each Chakra is related to certain aspects of the self "common Chakra parlance." For example the 1st Chakra is related to the physical body, the 2nd to the emotional self, the 3rd to the intellect, etc...

Harish Johari, in his book *Chakras, Energy Centers of Transformation (1976),* detailed not only the classical tantric information from the *Sat Cakra Nirupama (1544),* but also added his own take on the psychological "stages" of the Chakras. For example : the 1st Chakra personality is interested in survival, the 2nd in sex, 3rd in power, etc...

The modern vision we often have of the Chakras comes from *Nuclear Evolution* (1977) written by Dr.Christopher Hills, a scientist and philosopher (who would later become known for his idea to save starving humanity with spirulina).
He suggests that each Chakra corresponds to one of the seven colors of the spectrum. He also associates each Chakra and color with a particular personality type.
Although the psychological aspects of his theory did not really catch on, the idea of matching the seven Chakras with the seven colors of the spectrum was so compelling that just about every representation on the Chakras we can find on books since then show the Chakras in rainbow colors.

The most recent interpretations on the Chakras thus combine information from:
• *The Serpent Power*
• Teachings from Osho, Johari, Leadbeater, Brennan, Judith, Myss, etc...
• Hill's rainbow color schemata
• Various New Age themes involving healing, correspondences with crystals and gemstones, the musical scale, etc...
This combination constitutes what could be considered "Chakra Dogma". Numerous books, charts, artwork, t-shirts, massage kits, healing therapies, essential oil blends and more have been developed based on this amalgamated paradigm. However, we will soon see why matching the seven Chakras with the rainbow colors is not the most accurate thing to do.

Most recently, Dr.David Frawley delineates inner and outer Chakras in his book *Yoga and Ayurveda* (1999):
"One's Chakras can be closed on a spiritual level and yet one can be healthy, emotionally balanced, mentally creative, and successful in life. This depends upon outer, not inner Chakra functioning."
Actually, the so-called Chakra healers work with outer Chakras whereas Tantrics work with inner Chakras. We can access both through yoga but the inner Chakras can only be accessed by the yogi him/herself.
Modern interpretation of the Chakras seem to relate them mostly to the external personality and external body – these are the outer Chakras.
On the other hand, tantric Chakras are subtle faculties related to the subtle inner being – these are the inner Chakras. According to Tantra, the subtler self controls the coarser layers of being. In other words, our subtle minds can control our emotions and body, so it makes sense to work with inner Chakras.

6 LINKS BETWEEN THE PHYSICAL BODY, THE EMOTIONAL BODY AND THE CHAKRAS

In the physical body, one can associate each Chakra with nerve plexi and glands. These are the biological structures that interface with our psychological states.
Similarly, our psychological states influence the function of these structures.

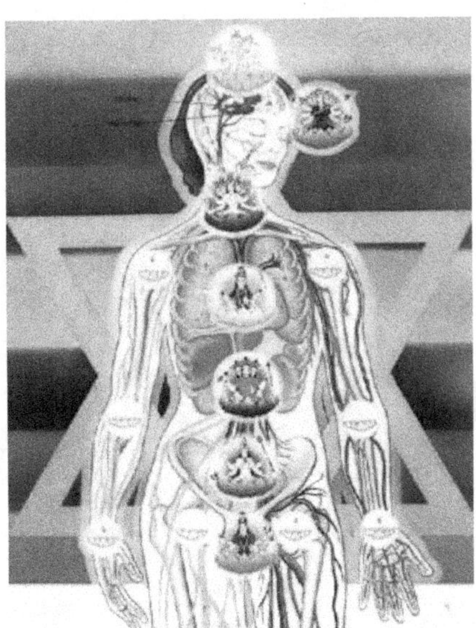

It is important here to emphasize the role of the gap junctions. Gap junctions are a linkage of two adjacent cells consisting of a system of channels extending across a gap from one cell to the other, allowing the passage of ions and small molecules. They coordinate the activity in many embryological processes and are more important neurologically at the embryologic stages – later chemical activity becomes more important. They synchronize endocrine secretions.

When the spine was developing, the neural fold cells used gap junctions. Therefore the spinal column has a lot of conductivity. Chakras can thus be seen as remnants of embryological organizing centers within the central nervous system (CNS).

As the embryo matures some of these cells migrate and become cells of the autonomous nervous system (ANS). The electrical connections still exist.

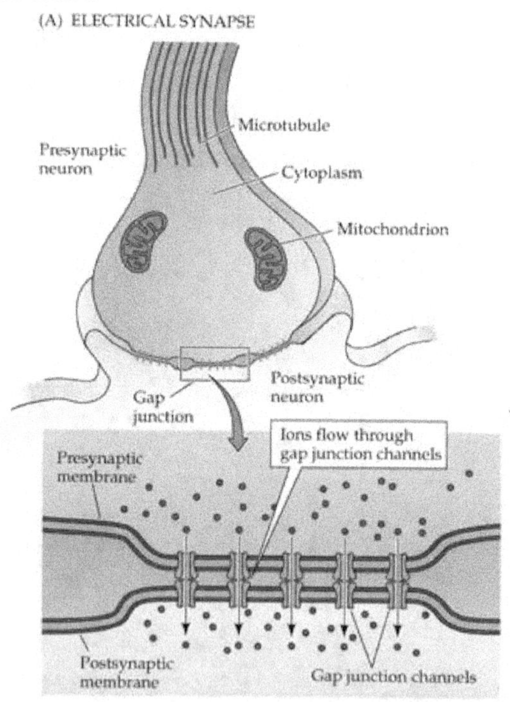

NEUROSCIENCE, Fourth Edition, Figure 5.1

Thus there are gap junction links between ANS cells and CNS cells. You can affect the CNS through the ANS because of these gap junction connections that were started embryonically.
Indeed, Chakra concentration points and asanas use the ANS to affect the CNS.

There is increasing research around the function of gap junctions. This research is suggestive of the existence and function of the Chakras. Gap junctions [would] create a channel all the way up the spine and provide a basis for the movement of the Kundalini – an electrical rather than chemical process.
Source: Richard W. Maxwell in *"The Physiological Foundation of Yoga Chakra Expression"*

There are no major nerve plexi associated with Ajna (6th Chakra) and Sahasrara (7th Chakra). However, the cranium bones and cartilage are formed from neural crest cells (the same stuff that forms the spine embryonically) and these bones retain subtle, energetic links to the CNS.

Chakras - Nerve Plexi Connections
7th   - none (cerebral cortex)
6th   - carotid plexus
5th   - pharyngeal plexus
4th   - cardiac and pulmonary plexi
3rd   - solar plexus
2nd   - lumbo-sacral plexus
1st   - coccygeal plexus

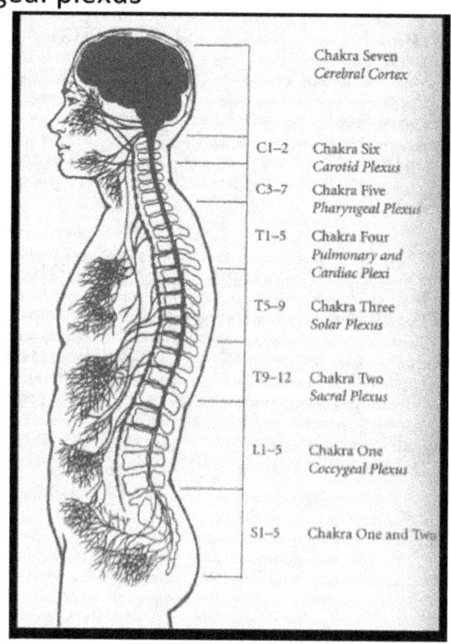

Chakras - Glands Connections

7th   - pineal
6th   - pituitary
5th   - thyroid and parathyroids
4th   - thymus
3rd   - adrenals and pancreas
2nd   - testes and ovaries
1st   - coccygeal bodies, urophysis remnants

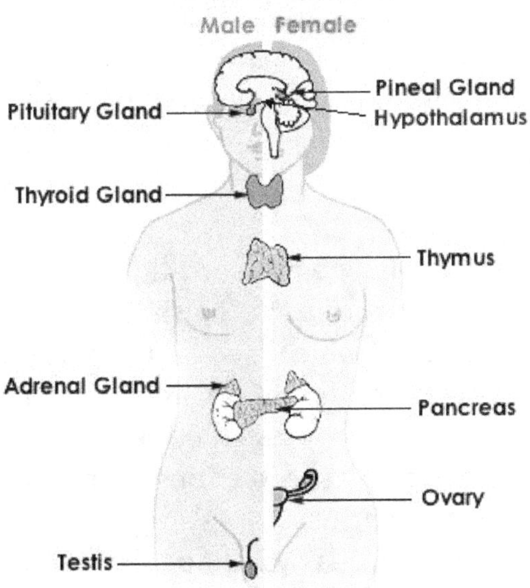

Still scientifically speaking, Dr. Valerie Hunt, a researcher at UCLA, found that there are high frequency vibrations emanating from the seven Chakras.

Candace Pert, who was a famous American pharmacologist who worked on neuropeptides, said that "...*there is a very close correspondence between the highest, most concentrated areas of enrichment of a certain neuropeptide and where the Chakras are classically supposed to be - there's a striking concordance. The seven centers actually correspond in places of enriched neuropeptide VIP (vasoactive intestinal peptide), which is an incredibly important neuropeptide, critical in regulating the neural immune switches between the brain and the immune system...*"

As for Hiroshi Motoyama, who was a parapsychologist who studied the links between body and mind, his research has shown that the energy systems in the body communicate via the medium of the fascia (the gelatinous "stuff" that exists around every structure in the body).
The Chakras energetically communicate with each other through the fascia via the subtle nadi system – primarily the ida, pingala and sushumna.

To summarize, we can say that Chakras are psycho-energetic. Through an understanding of cellular communication through gap junctions, we see that they are the way the body communicates electrically. Chakras and Nadis can communicate because of gap junctions.

From an endocrine viewpoint, secretions from glands create mental/emotional tendencies. In Sanskrit, these tendencies are called "vrttis" from "avit" which means "to rotate".
Vrttis effect the mind by the interaction of glandular secretions with brain systems which process emotion.
According to yoga theory, it is secretions from glands which create mental/emotional tendencies.
Indeed, through the nervous system part of the neuro-endocrine system, there is an instantaneous "state" created in the body/mind.

Yogis identified 50 main tendencies (Vrttis) associated with different glands in the body.
Each Chakra symbol (archetype) has a precise number of petals.
Each Vrtti is represented by one petal on the Chakra.
Each petal is inscribed with one of the 50 letters of the Sanskrit alphabet. These letters are the "acoustic roots" (fundamental sound vibrations) of the mental/emotional tendency.

The 7th Chakra, which is called Sahasrara (« The 1000 Petaled Lotus »), actually contains all the tendencies :
50 tendencies
x 2 (internal and external)
x 10 (motor and sensory organs)
= 1000 tendencies

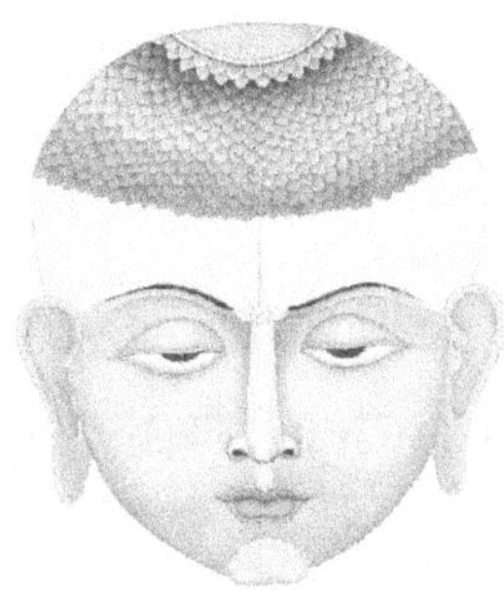

As P.R.Sarkar, an Indian yogi master and philosopher of the 20th century, said : *"In the human mind various thoughts are constantly emerging and dissolving. Behind these psychic phenomena are the underlying vrttis which are primarily related to the inborn sam'ska'ras of human beings. Propensities are formed according to one's inherent sam'ska'ras, and the expression and control of these propensities are dependent upon the various Chakras.*
The 50 main propensities of the human mind are expressed internally or externally through the vibrational expression of these Chakras. These vibrations cause hormones to be secreted from the glands, and the natural or unnatural expression of the propensities depends on the degree of normal or abnormal secretion of the hormones.
When these propensities can be expressed we say that the human mind is alive because the mind exists as long as the propensities are there. When the propensities are destroyed, however, the human mind loses its existence."

7 BALANCING THE CHAKRAS

In the 21st century western world, our thinking, even in spiritual, yoga or New Age communities, is mostly materialistic. We understand being and evolution as having a physical causality.
However, Eastern thinking structures define causality as spiritual. Therefore the deepest healing is only possible through spiritual practices.

According to Tantra, we can balance the Chakras by bringing the elements of our own Chakra system into balance with the cosmic forces of the universe.
Meditation on the color, shape, sound and energies of the element are techniques to help balance the Chakras.

As we have seen earlier, each Chakra is the microcosmic expression of one of the 5 cosmic element (see *Powers of the Tattvas*" - Woodroffe).
These elements are the "stuff" that makes up the expressed universe.

According to the Tantrics, the cosmic elements vibrate universally – vibrations create specific shapes, colors, and sounds.

To balance your Chakras, you must bring them into harmony with the cosmic vibrations of the universal elements.

Chakras are the way in which the universe organizes itself in you. They are the structure of the "drop" of Brahman.
As such, if you want to evolve, you must do intuitional work with the Chakras and the elements.

Some variations occur in the Tantric texts but globally here are the colors, shapes and sounds of the Chakras :

Chakra	Color	Shape	Sound
7th	No color	No shape	No sound
6th	No color	No shape	Tham or Om
5th	Iridescent	Many shapes	Ham
4th	Smoky green	Hexagon	Yam
3th	Red	Triangle	Ram
2nd	White	Crescent moon	Vam
1st	Gold	Square	Lam

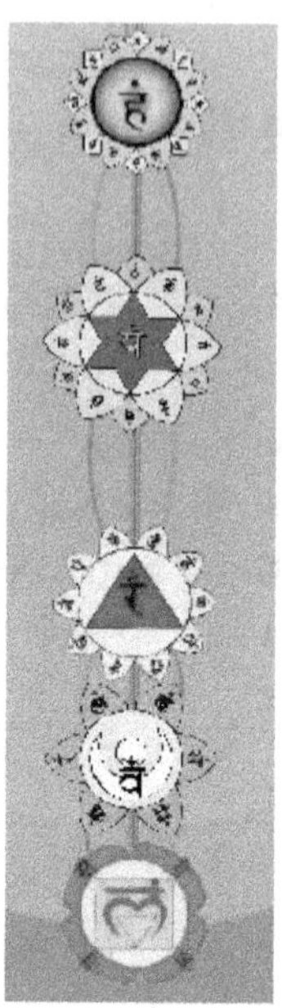

When your elements vibrate in harmony with the universe, your Chakras are balanced.
This is the practice of tantric yoga. For the yogi, attending to Chakra imbalance is the work of life.

Actually, Chakra "imbalances" mean you exist. According to the Tantrics the work of life is to deal with these imbalances as they arise.

Yoga is the Tantric way to balance the Chakras, with the help of :
- Meditation on Chakras
- Mudras (symbolic gestures)
- Chanting
- Diet and lifestyle
- Asanas (postures)
- Ethics (Yama and Niyama)
- Service

In order to shift the mind, you must influence the neuroendocrine system. This can be done by meditation, ideation, intention, therapy, drugs, etc...

The neuroendocrine system can also be influenced by asanas.

Repeating an asana puts a sustained and specific pressure on a gland, and pumps blood and lymphatic fluid through the gland and the tissue surrounding the gland. This is like "exercising" your glands. It has a tonifying/balancing effect on the body and the mind.

Repeating asanas sends subtle pulsations to the CNS. It also creates more functional neuromuscular pathways. These pathways create space in the structure to allow prana to flow through the nadis more freely. The mind is "freed up."

In addition pose repetition reinforces optimal movement patterns, builds muscle and lessens discomfort in the body.

For better results with asanas, you should :
• Bring the mind to the Chakra you are working on.
• Repeat the poses.
• Practice every 12 hours for maximum effect.
• A "clean" diet makes asanas more effective.

As we generally know now what the Chakras are, how they work and how to balance them, let us explore what they are and what they mean individually...

8   THE FIRST CHAKRA AND INDIVIDUAL POTENTIAL

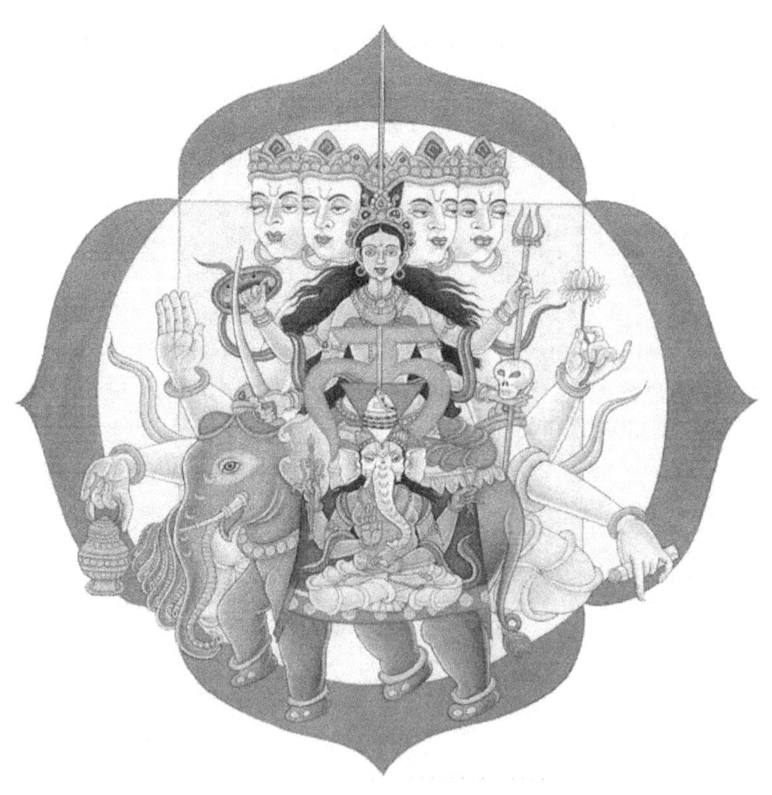

The 1st Chakra is called **Muladhara** which means "The Root Support". It is located at the same level as the base of the spine but in front of it.

As C.G.Jung wrote : *"Awakening the Kundalini means to separate the gods from the world so that they become active. From the standpoint of the gods, the world is less than child's play, it is merely a seed."*

Here are the archetypes of Muladhara:
- Element: Earth (Kshiti Tattva), the solid factor.
- Color: Golden
- Symbol: Square

As life is solid, firm and clear.

We also find:
- An inverted red triangle which represents the yoni, the fertile ground for consciousness to awaken and grow.
- A Shiva lingam which represents consciousness in itself.
- Airavata, a mystical elephant, which represents mundane, daily living, as the elephant is the "workhorse" of India and also the carrier of the Gods.
- Dakini, a female deity, who is fanged, brutal and scary. She represents the nasty part of ourselves that resists, that doesn't want to change.
- The youth Balbrahma. She represents potential, possibility, vision and idealism.

Muladhara has 4 petals, 4 Vrttis:
- Greatest bliss (paramananda)
- Innate bliss (sahajananda)
- Heroic bliss (virananda)
- Bliss of union (yogananda)

The petals represent the 4 human goals of existence (purusharthas):

- Physical desire (kama)
- Desire for psychic expansion (artha)
- Desire for social justice (dharma)
- Desire for spiritual freedom (moksha)

An imbalanced Muladhara would cause psycho-emotional issues related to these Vrttis. Mulhadara is responsible for the primary needs of survival: physical, mental and spiritual security and desire. If Mulhadara is well balanced, we are excited, we feel centered and anchored. Imbalanced, this Chakra can lead to an identity crisis and/or to feel like surviving rather than living. There is no known physical issue due to an imbalanced Muladhara but this Chakra might be linked to the water balance in the body.

The mantra of Muladhara is Lam (or Lung). His yantra is a yellow square. Prithvi mudra is its symbolic gesture:

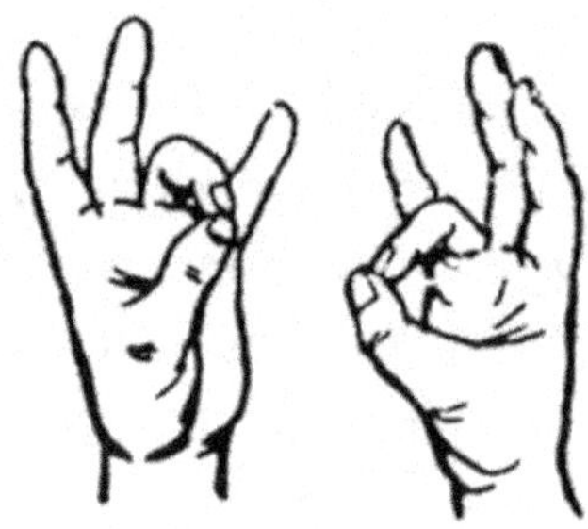

Balancing Muladhara can be done by doing asanas like inversions and pelvic floor work (Mulabandha), Bhavasana, Savasana, yoga nidra, mantra meditation (on the sound Lam) and meditation upon the following questions: « What am I besides this body? What am I besides all the labels I identify with? »

9 THE SECOND CHAKRA AND TRAUMA

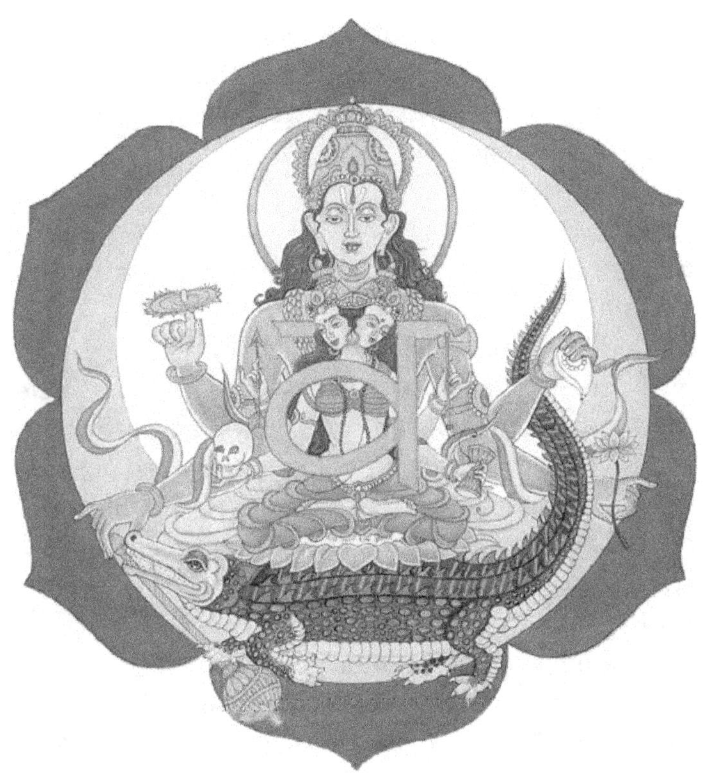

"Each Chakra is a whole world." - C.G.Jung

The 2nd Chakra is called **Svadhisthana**, « The One's Own Abode ». It is located at the level of the ovaries, in the lower abdomen. Svdhisthana is the Chakra which stocks all the traumas.

Here are the archetypes of Svadhisthana:
- Element: Water (*Api Tattva*), the liquid factor. Judith Lewis Herman, an American psychiatrist, researcher, teacher, and author who has focused on the understanding and treatment of incest and traumatic stress, says about a traumatized person that she is: « *icy cold inside and my surfaces are without integument, as if I am flowing and spilling and not held together any more. Fear grips me and I lose the sensation of being present. I am gone.*"
- Color: Moonlight on water (white)
- Symbol: Crescent Moon, which is the symbol of the water element. It represents fresh start, rebirth, awakening and victory over death.

We also find:
- Makara – the water monster. Makara can represent the trauma.
  As said by J.L.Herman, "*The ordinary response to atrocities is to banish them from consciousness. Certain violations of the social compact are too terrible to utter aloud: this is the meaning of the word* unspeakable."
  In One's Own Abode "*Traumatized people feel utterly abandoned, utterly alone, cast out of the human and divine systems of care and protection that sustain life.*" - J.D.Herman
- Varuna – The God of Water.
- Rakini, a female deity, who is fierce and drunk.
- Vishnu, a male deity, who is the Preserver, the Rescuer.

Svadhisthana has 6 petals, 6 Vrttis:
- Indifference, disdain (*Avajna*)

- Stupor (*Murcha*)
- Indulgence, substance abuse (*Prashraya*)
- No confidence, distrust (*Avishvasa*)
- Fear, helplessness (*Sarvanasha*)
- Cruelty (*Krurata*)

Svadhistana being the Chakra which retains traumas, we will briefly explore how these Vrttis are linked to traumas.

- Sarvanasha is the fear of complete annihilation, helplessness. *"A wide array of animal experiments show that when high levels of adrenaline and other stress hormones are circulating, memory traces are deeply imprinted."* - Herman
Herman also exposes that children who are frequently abused dissociate in order to cope and that when dissociation goes too far, the experience is one of complete disconnection from others and disintegration of the self.
• The yogis would call dissociation Murcha.
• The yogis would call the complete disconnection *Sarvanasha*, a sense of complete self-annihilation.
"While the mind usually shuts down during a traumatizing experience, the bodily sensations associated with immobilization and helplessness carry the memories of having absolutely no control over the outcome of your life: the fate of trauma survivors is lived out in heartbreak and gut-wrenching sensations." – E. Hooper and D. Emerson
Herman states that profound dissociative states with a sense of unbearable agitation precede a need to self mutilate and that this mutilation provides a relief from the unbearable sensations in the body. Self-mutilation being basically a self soothing behavior. This kind of self-mutilation is an expression of Sarvanasha.

- Murcha can be translated into « stupor », *"As in the Greek myth of Medusa, the human confusion that may ensue when we stare death in the face can turn us to stone. We may literally freeze in*

fear, which will result in the creation of traumatic symptoms." –
Peter A.Levine, American trauma specialist and therapist.

- Prashraya is indulgence or substance abuse. *"The risk of heavy
drinking, self-reported alcoholism, and marrying an alcoholic were
increased twofold to fourfold by the presence of multiple ACEs,
regardless   of   parental   alcoholism."*
(http://www.ncbi.nlm.nih.gov/pubmed/12201379?dopt=Abstract
)
*"Alcohol makes the body feel safe. Until you find an alternative
way, you can't quit drinking... But we can do something to change
the internal experience without alcohol."* – Bessel van der Kolk
(Danish clinician, researcher and teacher in the area of
posttraumatic stress).

- Avishvasa can be translated into « no confidence » or
« distrust ». We can link it to hypervigilence. *"Few symptoms
provide more insight into a traumatic experience than
hypervigilance. Hypervigilance is a direct and immediate
manifestation of hyperarousal, which is the intial response to
threat. Its effect on the orienting response is particularly
debilitating, setting the traumatized individual up for an ongoing
experience of fear, paralysis and victimization."* – P.A.Levine

- Avajna is indifference, disdain. *"I have always just numbed out.
That way, I don't feel anything inside. I don't feel my own self, and
I don't feel any connection to other people... If the feelings are too
strong to numb them, I will take drugs or get drunk to guarantee I
get rid of them."*, testimony gathered by David Berceli,
international expert in the areas of trauma intervention and
conflict resolution.

- Krurata is cruelty. Some years ago, a Marine Lance Corporal in
Texas, returned from three back-to-back tours of duty in Iraq, and
allegedly suffering from PTSD, breaks into his former girlfriend's
home, stabs her to death and then waits, *"covered with blood and*

looking dazed", in the parking lot for police to arrive and arrest him.

Besides its links with traumas, Svadhisthana rules the "common sense" and self-confidence. An imbalanced Svadhistana can lead to neglect of others, to make actions of cruelty (towards oneself, animals or other human beings), to abuse hard drugs, or to feel down, depressed, without possibility to resurface.
An imbalanced Svadhisthana also leads to physical disorders like: Reproductive problems, menstrual dysfunction, polycystic ovary syndrome, certain cancers in the pelvic area and osteoporosis.

More will be said in chapter 14 on yoga and traumas. Chapter 15 will discuss yoga and addictions.

The mantra of Svadhisthana is Vam (or Wung). His yantra is a white crescent moon. Varuna mudra is its symbolic gesture:

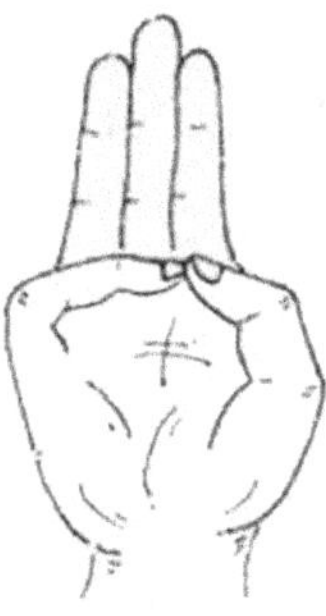

We can balance Svadhisthana and address traumas at the same time with yoga. This can be done by: Doing asanas which produce shaking (like holding Utkatasana for a long period of time) and sweating, primal pranayamas (like Breath of Joy, exhaling through the mouth, etc...), vocalizing (Oms, chanting during asanas), practicing all types of hip openers, and practicing poses wich require hands on the earth. Yoga Nidra and deep relaxation will help too, as well as compassion (*Metta*) and Tonglen meditations. Eyes can be opened during meditation.

ASIDE ON TRAUMAS

I think it is important to make an aside about traumas as an ending of this chapter. We have seen how Svadhisthana is linked to traumas and how to address them. But what are they?

A trauma can be defined as:
1. A serious injury or shock to the body, as from violence or an accident.
2. An emotional wound or shock that creates substantial, lasting damage to the psychological development of a person, often leading to neurosis.
3. An event or situation that causes great distress and disruption. The word com from the Greek *tere* "to rub, to turn".

Post-Traumatic Stress Disorder (PTSD) is an anxiety disorder that can occur after a traumatic event. A PTSD diagnosis can occur when a person experienced a traumatic event which involved actual threatened death or serious injury or the threat to the physical integrity of self or others.
In PTSD, these four symptoms are present:
1. The traumatic event was very threatening and was followed by intense fear and/or helplessness.
2. The event is re-experienced in a number of ways.
3. There is a persistent avoidance of stimuli associated with the trauma and a numbing of general responsiveness.
4. There are persistent symptoms of increased arousal including insomnia, irritability, difficulties concentrating, etc...
Symptoms of PTSD may include: Flashbacks, nightmares and sleep problems, depression, emotional detachment or numbness, easily startled, irritability, aggressive feelings, anxiety and substance abuse.

Statistically, we know that approximately 7.7 million American adults age 18 and older, or about 3.5 percent of people in this age group in a given year, have PTSD. We also know that 3.6 days of work impairment per month are associated with PTSD. This translates to an annual productivity loss in excess of $3 billion.

Traumas can come from 2 different origins:
• Acute/Shock: Crime, experiencing or witnessing violence, natural disasters, car accidents, rescue work, etc...
• Complex/Developmental: Child abuse, neglect, abandonment, having alcoholic/drug addicted parents, etc...

We can predict the probability of a complex/developmental trauma to occur with the help of the Adverse Childhood Experiences (ACE). ACEs are:
1. Recurrent physical abuse
2. Recurrent emotional abuse
3. Contact sexual abuse
4. An alcohol and/or drug abuser in the household
5. An incarcerated household member
6. Living with someone who is chronically depressed, mentally ill, institutionalized, or suicidal
7. Mother is treated violently
8. One or no parents
9. Emotional or physical neglect
If a person gets 4 or more ACEs, there are:
• 240 percent greater risk of hepatitis
• 390 percent greater risk of COPD
• 240 percent greater risk of STDs
• Two times more likely to smoke
• 12 times more likely to attempt suicide
• 7 times more likely to be alcoholics
• 10 times more likely to inject street drugs
• More likely to be violent, have more marriages, broken bones, drug prescriptions, depression, auto-immune diseases, cancer, heart disease, liver disease, obesity and work absences.

Indeed, you have a greater chance of developing PTSD if you have been traumatized as a child. We all will experience life and death situations but those with more ACEs are more likely to develop PTSD, people with fewer ACEs are more neurologically resilient.

As we have seen earlier, traumas leave marks in the body. *"...a common denominator of all traumas is an alienation and disconnection from the body and a reduced capacity to be present in the here and now."* – P.A.Levine, in *Overcoming Trauma through Yoga.* *"The emotional pain we carry within us isn't just in our heads. It's etched in our muscles."* – D.Berceli, in *Trauma Releasing Exercises.*

With an unresolved trauma, the body is stuck in the past and bodily sensations are often painful or unbearable. It is to escape the sensations in their bodies that people turn to drugs, alcohol or other self-destructive behaviors.

10 THE THIRD CHAKRA AND HARNESSING THE ENERGY

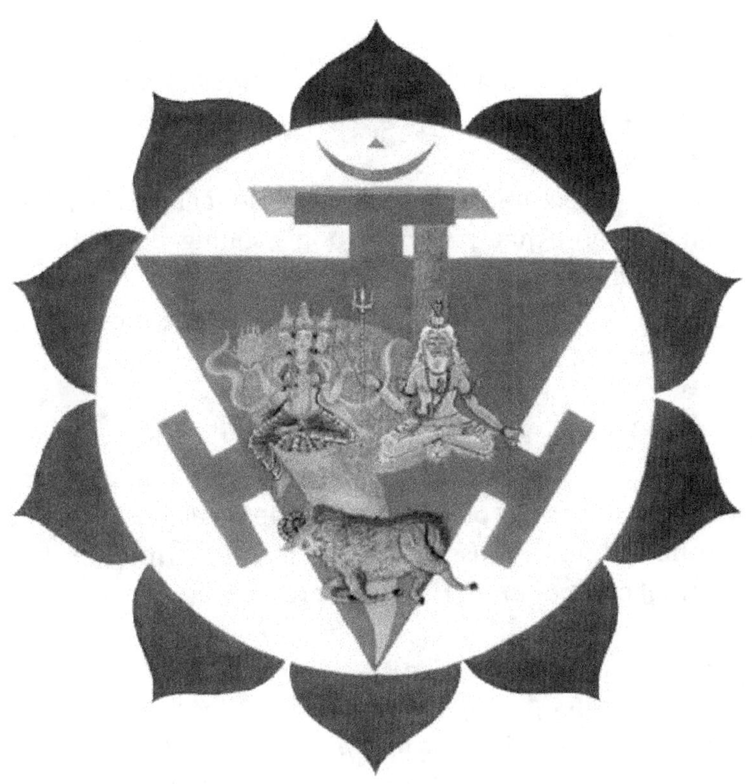

The third Chakra is called **Manipura** which means « The City of Jewels ». It is located between the solar plexus (which innervates the stomach, liver, gallbladder, spleen, kidney, small intestine, and the ascending and transverse colon) and the lumbar plexus. Its corresponding glands are the adrenals glands and the pancreas.

It is a place of great energetic wealth, the place where we can mine energy.

Here are the archetypes of Manipura:
- Element: Fire (*Tejas tattva*), the luminous factor
- Color: Red
- Symbol: Triangle (The triangle "flips up" when the Chakra is activated.)

We also find:
- A ram. As for Jung: *"It is now a sacrificial animal, and it is a relatively small sacrifice... The smaller sacrifice of the passions."*
- Lakini, a female deity, who is unselfconsciously bingeing on rice and meat, some blood running down her throat and sari.
- Rudra, a male deity, who wants your sacrifice and makes you cry. He is unselfconscious too.

Because of the fire element, Tantra says that Manipura is the place where we convert food into energy, the place of intense emotions and the place of alchemical transformation. Alchemy being the process of personal transformation. It needs two essential components: Heat and pressure...

Manipura has 10 petals, 10 Vrttis:
- Shyness, shame (*lajja*)
- Sadistic tendencies (*pishunata*)
- Envy (*iirsa*)
- Inertia, laziness, sleepiness (*susupti*)
- Melancholy, depression (*visada*)

- Irritability, peevishness (*kasaya*)
- Craving, yearning for power (*trsna*)
- Infatuation, blind attachment (*moha*)
- Hatred, revulsion (*ghrna*)
- Fear (*bhaya*)

Manipura is thus responsible for the strength that allows us to move forward, it is pure courage. We are therefore more playful, more motivated, more combative if Manipura is balanced.

Besides these psycho-emotional dysfunctions, an imbalanced Manipura can cause physical disorders like: Adrenal fatigue/exhaustion, diabetes, obesity, metabolic syndrome, Addisons and Cushings diseases.

The mantra of Manipura is Ram (or Rung). His yantra is a red triangle. Agni mudra is its symbolic gesture:

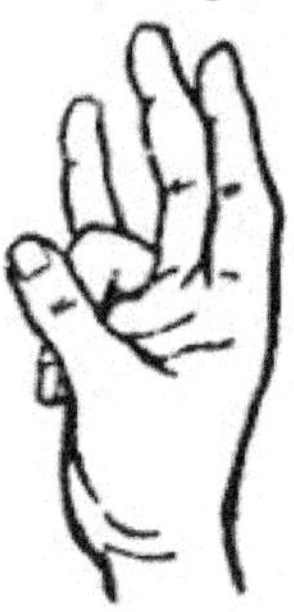

Balancing Manipura can be done following two axes:
• Transformation: Via "Agni" practices like Uddhiyana, Agnisara, Nauli and Mayurasana/Peacock pose (for detoxifying and strengthening), forward folds (for calming excited digestion and for dealing with anger, irritability and stress), back bends (for strengthening weak digestion, lessening fear and depression, and increasing strength and courage), and twists (for detoxifying).
• Releasing Neurotic Habits: With the help of cognitive practices like focusing on the opposite or focusing on the inner light ; mantra, visualizations (*bhavana*), service (*seva, tapas*) and community (*satsanga*).

11   THE FOURTH CHAKRA AND SELF-UNDERSTANDING

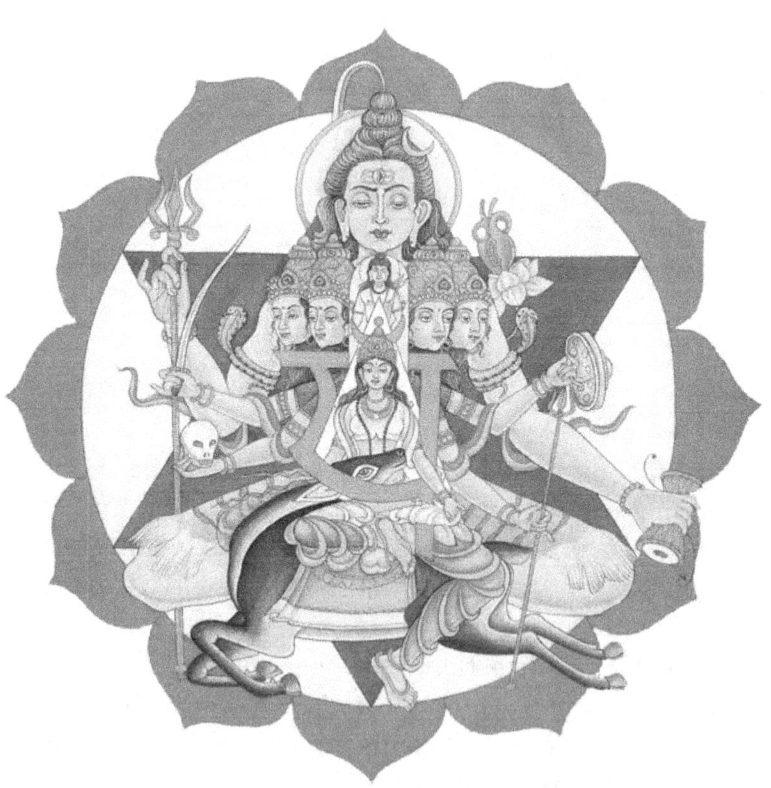

The 4th Chakra is called **Anahata** which means « The Unstruck ».
It is located at the level of the cardiac plexus (the cardiac plexus is

a plexus of nerves situated at the base of the heart that innervate the heart. It is divided into a superficial part, which lies in the concavity of the aortic arch and a deep part, between the aortic arch and the trachea. These are closely connected).
Its corresponding endocrine gland is the thymus.

For Jung, Anahata is the unattackable. It is the place where we lay down boundaries.

Here are the archetypes of Anahata:
- Element: Air (*Bhutta Tattva*), the aerial factor
- Color: Grayish green
- Symbol: 6 pointed star

We also find:
- A gazelle (antelope/deer), a free animal which represents the fact that the passions, having been controlled, are free to express themselves. It is freedom as a result of practice, discipline and self control.
  Its spiraled horns now move upward rather than spiraling back into the self (like those of the ram) and causing destruction.
- Kakini, a female deity, who is the Shakti depicted as a beautiful Goddess for the first time. She is offering the mudra of courage and fearlessness (*Virabhaya*).
- Ishana, a male deity, is the Compassionate One who represents knowing compassion and who has Christ-like wisdom and love.
  The water flowing from his head is the expression of the mantra *So Ham* « I am that » and the snakes coiled around his body represent the passions, which he has tamed. That is why Jospeh Campbell says: *"Parents are the heros of the Heart Chakra."*

Anahata has 12 petals, 12 Vrttis:
- Hope (*Asha*)

- Anxiety (*Cinta*)
- Effortfulness (*Cesta*)
- Love and attachment (*Mamata*)
- Vanity, arrogance (*Dambha*)
- Conscience, discrimination (*Viveka*)
- Psychic depression (*Vikalatah*)
- Ego (*Ahamkara*)
- Greed (*Lolata*)
- Deception (*Kapatah*)
- Argumentativeness, tendency to debate (*Vitarka*)
- Repentance (*Anutapa*)

Anahata is responsible for the feelings of hope, love and compassion. If Anahata is unbalanced, it is impossible to express deep feelings like joy.
Besides these psycho-emotional dysfunctions, an imbalanced Anahata can cause physical disorders like: Certain heart issues, certain cancers and immune system issues.

The mantra of Anahata is Yam (or Yung). His yantra is a green 6 branches star, an hexagon (which is, indeed, the inside of the star) or a circle. Vayu mudra is its symbolic gesture:

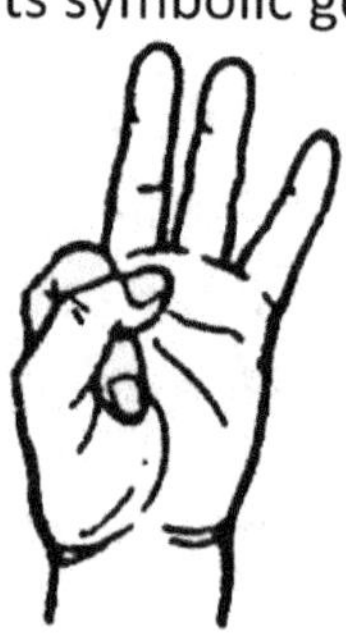

Balancing Anahata can be done working working on 3 axes:
• Boundaries: Meditation practices focused on the heart, longer inhale pranayamas. Ethics (Yamas and Niyamas). Practicing limits and decision making.

• Sense of self: Meditations on the heart Chakra, meditation of compassion (*Metta*).
• Critical thinking and ethical decision making (Yamas and Niyamas).
All asanas working on backbends are beneficial for Anahata.

ASIDE ON THE VECTOR EQUILIBRIUM AND THE TORE

New aside here about the Buckminster Fuller's Vector Equilibrium. Buckminster Fuller was an American architect, systems theorist, author, designer, and inventor. He published more than 30 books, coining or popularizing terms such as "Spaceship Earth", ephemeralization, and synergetic. The Vector Equilibrium would be the way that nature organizes energy.
Its shape is uncannily similar to that which the yogis called the heart Chakra.

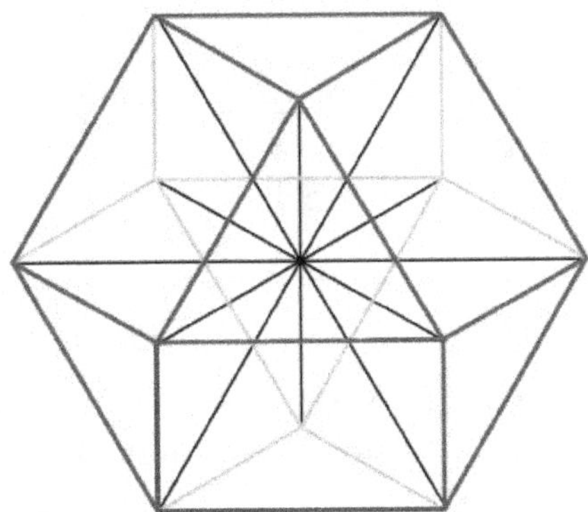

"The Vector Equilibrium is the anywhere, anywhen, eternally regenerative event inceptioning an evolutionary accommodation and will never be seen by man in any physical experience. Yet it is the frame of evolvement." – Buckminster Fuller.
"Equilibrium between positive and negative is zero... Zero pulsation in the Vector Equilibrium is the nearest approach we will ever know to eternity and God: The zero phase of conceptual integrity inherent in the positive and negative asymmetries that propagate the differentials of consciousness." – Buckminster Fuller.

"Vector equilibrium is a balanced destination of the spirit's devotional noble pursuit." – Buckminster Fuller.
Actually, Anahata's shape mirrors the Vector Equilibrium. You can notice a hexagon, a hexagram and a circle/sphere (toroid energy). Twelve radii/petals are also emanating from the center.
The sphere is of crucial importance here because, according to the HeartMath Institute, the human heart generates an energy field shaped like a torus. *"The heart generates by far the largest rhythmic electromagnetic field produced in the body. We've found that if we look at the spectrum analysis of the magnetic field created by the heart, the emotional information is coded and modulated into those fields."* – Rollin McCraty, Director of Research, HeartMath Institute

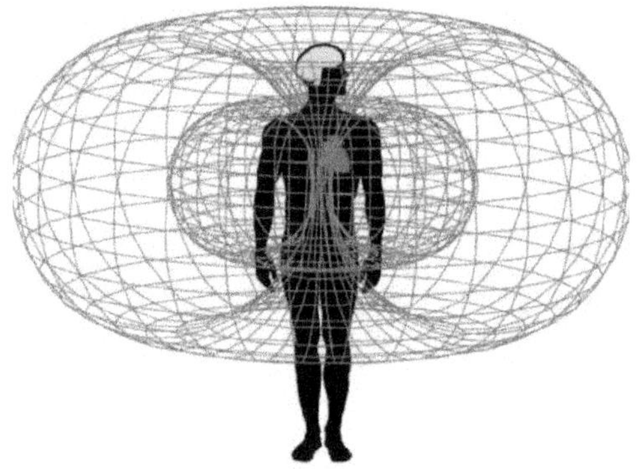

"By learning to shift our emotions, thus changing the information we're encoding into those magnetic fields affecting the heart, we can impact those around us." – Rollin McCraty, Director of Research, HeartMath Institute
We are talking here about something called mindsight. *"Mindsight"* is a term coined by Dr. Dan Siegel (an American psychiatrist and interpersonal neurobiologist) to describe our human capacity to perceive the mind of the self and others. It is a powerful lens through which we can understand our inner lives with more clarity, integrate the brain, and enhance our relationships with others.
Siegel research has shown that the gut, heart, and lungs all have neural networks that seek to communicate with the brain. When we attend to our Chakras, we move towards personal integration.

12 THE FIFTH CHAKRA AND SELF-ACTUALIZATION

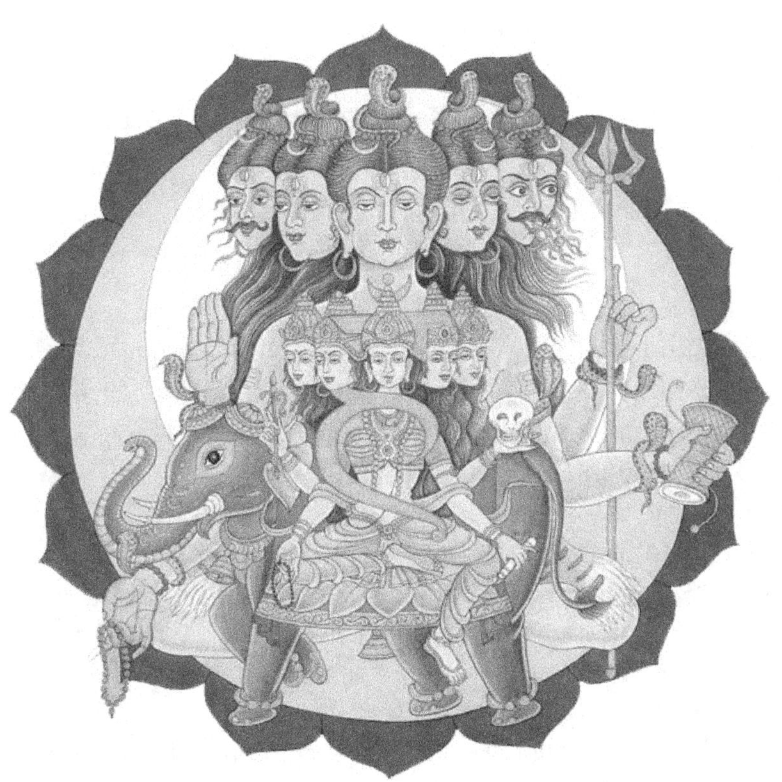

The 5th Chakra is called **Vishuddha** which means « The Pure » or « Purifying ». It is the place where impurities, distinctions and

boundaries dissolve. It is the bridge between the body and the mind. It is located between the cervical plexus and the pharyngeal plexus (which is formed by branches of the glossopharyngeal, vagus, and sympathetic nerves and which supplies the muscles and mucous membrane of the pharynx, palate and other parts of the throat).
Its corresponding glands are the thyroid and the parathyroids.

Carl Jung wrote: *"If I should succeed – and I hope I shall not – in taking all of you up to Vishuddha, you would certainly complain, you would stifle, you would not be able to breathe any longer, because there is nothing you could possibly breathe. It is ether. In reaching Vishuddha you reach the airless space where there is no earthly chance for the ordinary individual to breathe."*

Here are the archetypes of Vishuddha:
- Element: Ether (*Akasha Tattva*), the ethereal factor, which represents the realm between the worlds, the still point (*kumbhaka*)
- Color: None or all, like oil on water
- Symbol: None or all

We also find:
- Airavata, represented as a white elephant. It symbolizes the fact that all animals instincts have been purified. The realm of self has transcended the physical. The (elephantine) power is now purely in the psychic realm. It also represents the power of manifesting ideas.
- Shakini, a female deity, who is here the embodiment of purity and peace. She has 5 heads. This represents the control over the 5 elements and the 5 senses. She is the bestower of *Siddhis*, the powers. She holds a noose and a skull to show that you are not finished yet...
- Panchavaktra Shiva, a male deity, who has 5 heads too. He can see in all directions, he is omniscient. He is the combination of all other Shivas. The Kundalini dances on his head, controlled. It shows that everything is Self, nothing is outside.

Vishuddha is the abode of Shiva, the Lord of the Aesthetic. It is the abode of art, music, dance, etc... all that which expresses experience beyond words. Creativity and self-expression, are accessed through this Chakra.

Vishuddha has 16 petals, 16 Vrttis:
- Vibrancy, do tone, peacock (*Sadaja*)
- Relieving, re tone, bull, ox (*Rsabha*)
- Quieting, mi tone, goat (*Gandhara*)
- Peaceful, fa tone, horse (*Madhyama*)
- Joyful, sol tone, cuckoo (*Painchama*)
- Sweetness, donkey, la (*Dhaevata*)
- Tender longing, elephant, ti tone (*Nisada*)
- Root sound of creation/preservation/dissolution (*Om*)
- Root sound of rising Kundalini (*Hum*)
- Putting theory into practice, root sound of activation (*Phat*)
- Expression of mundane knowledge, root sound of physical welfare (*Vaosat*)
- Welfare in the subtler sphere, root sound of psychic welfare (*Vasatha*)
- Pious resolve, root sound of noble purpose, universal welfare (*Svaha*)
- Root sound of surrender to the Supreme (*Namah*)
- Root sound of repulsive poisonous expression (*Visa*)
- Root sound of sweet expression, attraction (*Amrta*)

Vishuddha causes all kinds of communication problems such as stuttering, excessive communication, mythomania, fear of public speaking, aphasia, etc... Vishuddha also causes the inability to really listen to others.
Besides these psycho-emotional dysfunctions, an imbalanced Vishuddha can cause physical disorders like: Thyroid diseases, osteoporosis, certain cancers in the area and hearing problems.

The mantra of Vishuddha is Ham (or Hung). His yantra is multi-shaped and multi-colored. Akasha mudra is its symbolic gesture:

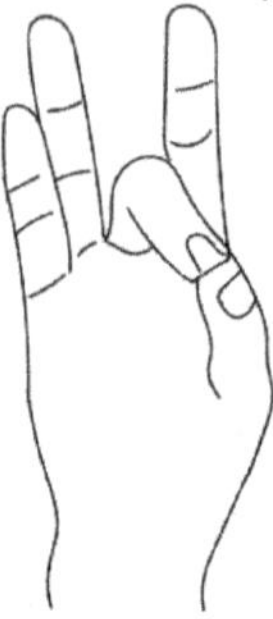

Balancing Vishuddha can be done working on:
• Self-Expression: Kirtan, chanting, art, journaling and personal development work.
• Self-Actualization: Mantra meditation, yoga poses with Jalandhara Bandha/Chin Lock, yoga poses which work on the neck area (Matsyasana/Fish pose, Halasana/Plow pose, Chakrasana/Wheel pose, …), service and devotional practices.

13 THE SIXTH AND SEVENTH CHAKRAS AND HUMAN POTENTIAL

a. Ajna

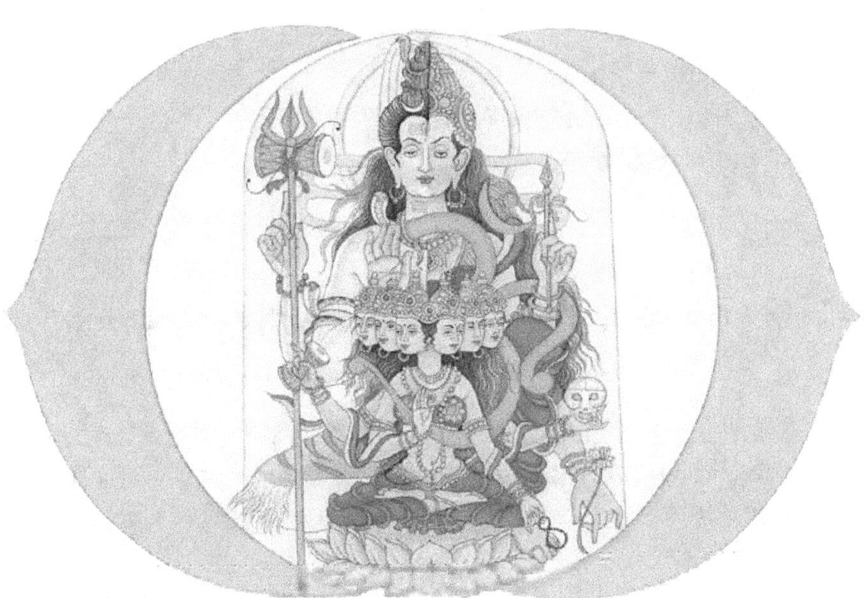

The 6th Chakra is Called **Ajna**, « The Command Center ». It corresponds to the hypothalamus and to the pituitary gland.

Ajna is beyond the physical: Elements, color, sound and shape are not relevant because this Chakra does not exist in the mundane realm. Ajna belongs to a purely psychic realm. For this reason there is no animal archetypes anymore.

Here are the archetypes of Ajna:
- Hakini, a female deity, who is completely pure and glowing like the moon. She has the control over the Kundalini (she is holding the snake). She is also holding the Amrita – the nectar of bliss (hormones). The Shakti has softened, she doesn't have to be so fierce here, most of the work has already been done.
- Ardhanarishvara, a deity, who is the merging of the male and female principles. It represents the dissolution of opposites.
- Om (ॐ), standing for the triangle symbolism (*Trikona*). 3 Gods: Brahma, Vishnu and Shiva. 3 Qualities (*Gunas*): Purity (*Sattva*), Desire (*Rajas*) and Inertia (*Tamas*). 3 Bodies: Physical, Mental and Spiritual.

Ajna has 2 petals, 2 Vrittis:
- All spiritual knowledge (*para*)
- All mundane knowledge (*apara*)

An imbalanced Ajna can cause focusing and memory problems. It can also cause disillusions and disappointments.
Physically, an imbalanced Ajna can cause growth disorders, headaches, hallucinations, eye problems and insomnia.

Ajna is what is often called the 3rd Eye. It is pure intuition, which is beyond the intellect. It represents spiritual awareness and is the place where nadis (energy pathways) merge, where duality dissolves.

The mantra of Ajna is Om (or Thung or Tham). It has no yantra. Hakini Mudra is its symbolic gesture:

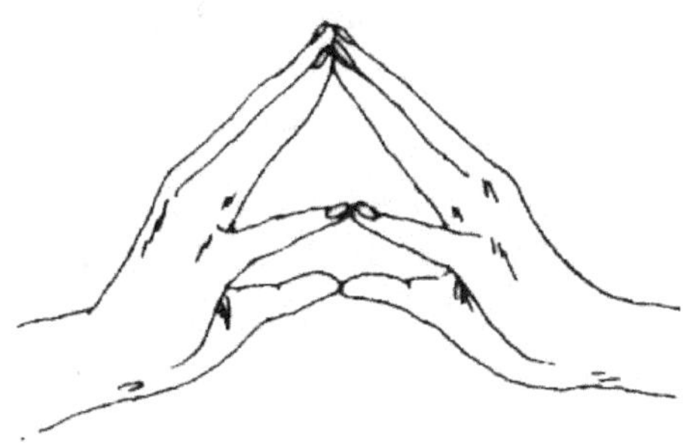

b. Sahasrara

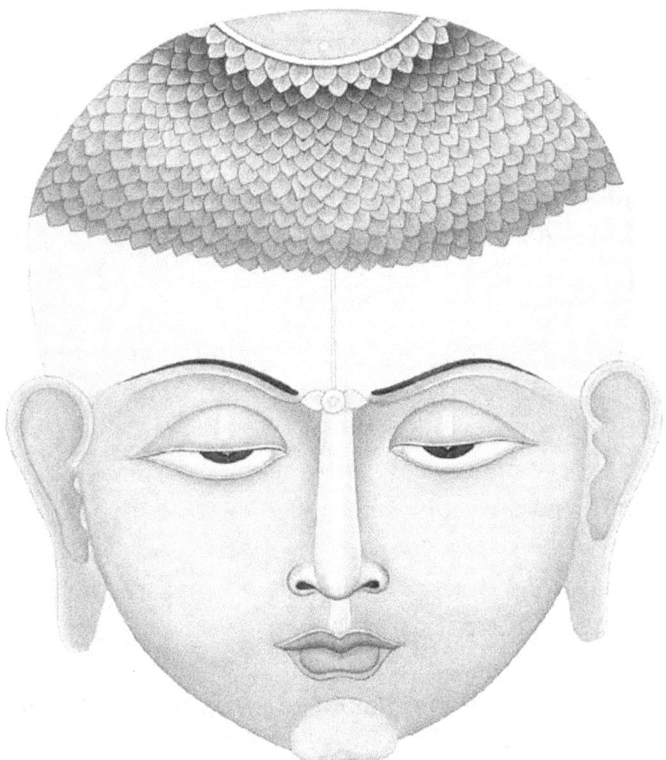

The 7th Chakra is called **Sahasrara**, « The One Thousand-Petaled Lotus ». It is located in the cerebral cortex.Its corresponding gland is the pineal (also called epiphysis).

"To speak about the lotus of the thousand petals above, the Sahasrara center, is quite superfluous because that is merely a philosophical concept with no substance to us whatever; it is beyond any possible experience. In Ajna, there is still the experience of the self that is apparently different from the object, God. But in Sahasrara one understands that is not different, and so the next conclusion would be that there is no object, no god, nothing but Brahman. There is no experience because it is one, it is without a second. It is dormant, it is not, and therefore it is nirvana. This is an entirely philosophical concept, a mere logical conclusion from the premises before. It is without practical value for us." – Carl Jung, *The Psychology of Kundalini Yoga*

As for the archetypes of Sahasrara, it has no element or symbols, only petals. It is extra-cerebral: The energy of the Sahasrara is created by brain systems, but it actually exists slightly above the crown of the head. Its petals represent all the possibilities of human expression, merging into Oneness. Sahasrara is beyond description, purely experiential.

An imbalanced Sahasrara can lead to confusion, amnesia, spiritual addiction, learning difficulties, exacerbated materialism, limited beliefs or spiritual skepticism.
Physically an imbalanced Sahasrara can can lead to neurological problems, migraines or insomnia.

For all the reasons seen above, there is no mantra, no yantra and no mudra corresponding to Sahasrara.

Ajna and Sahasrara can be balanced with the help of the same techniques, working on:
• Equanimity and deep connection via Dhyana (contemplative meditation), kirtan and devotional practices.
• Self-Realization via Dhyana (contemplative meditation) and retreats/residential programs.

14   RESTING THE CHAKRAS

Statistics show us that we are living mental health crises:
- 1 in 4 adults has a diagnosable mental disorder, 1 in 17 have a Serious Mental Illness (SMI).
- Mental illness health care cost nearly $60 billion - equivalent to the cost of cancer care.
- Untreated mental illness costs the United States more than $100 billion a year.
- About 15 percent of the U.S. population can be considered "problem drinkers" !
- Nine percent of Americans over the age of 12 are abusing or dependent upon illicit drugs.
- By 2030 - Cardiovascular disease, chronic respiratory disease, cancer, diabetes, and mental health will represent a cumulative output loss of $47 trillion – roughly 75% of the global GDP in 2010.

We can conclude that our paradigms of human existence are inadequate. Consciousness studies represent the frontier of a deeper understanding of what it means to be human. Hopefully, Chakras are an entry point to understanding consciousness. Nerve plexi and glands are associated with each Chakra. These are the biological structures that interface with our psycho-physical states and can affect those states.

We must remember that we have the capacity to influence our Chakras and therefore our health outcomes.

Chakras are a reflection of the Tantric finding: Body manifests from mind and mind from spirit. They help us understand both ontology and the mechanisms of health from a non-materialistic perspective.

15   YOGA AND TRAUMAS

"Every trauma, whether it occurs in a physiological, cognitive, emotional or interpersonal form, affects the physical body. The healing of trauma begins in the body.
Since the body is an accurate history book of our experiences in life, it is essential that we include the body in the healing process." – D.Berceli, PhD. Trauma Researcher, in *Trauma Releasing Exercises*.

When threatened, we naturally curl up into a fetal position. This is the "universal position" of trauma which protects the face and all of the internal organs.
The psoas muscles are the primary flexor muscles that contract - the "sentinels" that protect us from harm. To heal the consequences of trauma, and some think the trauma itself, we can help the body relax the psoas tension with yoga postures and other practices.

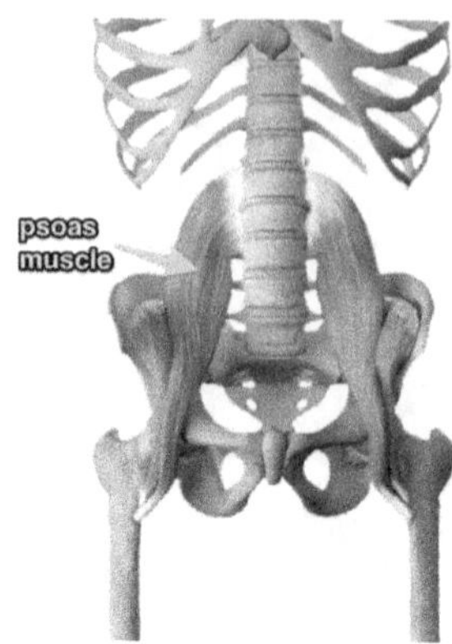

When we are traumatized, we are separated from ourselves, from our bodies, as well as from the present moment.
Yoga can mean "union" or integration of the body, mind and spirit and/or "union" of the self with a higher power. The practices of yoga are thus intended to help bring the disparate parts of ourselves back together.

Yoga has the power to heal traumas by working on:
- Body: Yoga offers postures and breathing practices to help heal the body.
- Mind: Yoga offers grounding, orienting and visualization practices, and yoga nidra, as well as the emphasis on community (*Satsanga*) and ethics (*Yamas* and *Niyamas*) to help heal the mind.
- Spirit: Yoga practices like meditation, kirtan and mindfulness help soothe and expand the spirit.

We can briefly study here how Yoga helps in healing traumas. Actually, the fight, flight or freeze mechanisms (natural reactions to stress) are easy to turn on and hard to turn off. Moreover, post-traumatic stress disorders result when we don't have an outlet to release traumas from the body.
We then can mitigate the hypothalamic-pituitary-adrenal axis activation and dampen down the effects of trauma induced agitation (especially the release of cortisol, the stress hormone) by activating

the relaxation response through deep relaxation and restorative yoga poses and practices like Savasana or Yoga Nidra.

We also have to work on the psoas and other flexor muscles which must release their contraction.

Holding poses, like Utkatasana/Chair pose, until the body starts to tremor (neurogenic tremoring) can also help "unfreeze" the trauma. We will see why later.

Another yogic approach is recreating the trauma position in a safe environment. This helps the body to release the muscle tension and allow the body to understand that it can release the experience of trauma.

Furthermore, Yoga helps to stay out of the past, into the present. It is self-induced, self-regulated – through mindfulness, breathing and postures. It is also non-judgmental, non-threatening and non-competitive.

Jodi Carey, a famous yoga teacher from the Trauma Center of Boston, says about Yoga that: « *Asana is a powerful tool that acts as a system of neuromuscular re-patterning that can teach the entire organism how to re-organize itself.* »

Yoga can be seen as a Public Health Strategy. Because so many people have experienced trauma in their lives (7.7 million American adults age 18 and older, or about 3.5 percent of people in this age group in a given year, have PTSD), trauma is a major public health issue. So, the accessibility of yoga within and outside of a professional context makes it an important community health strategy.

Yoga can be seen as transformational. Indeed, as David Berceli says: « *Because the traumatic experience is outside our present worldview and ability to process logically, it seems completely overwhelming and unbearable.*

However it is precisely because it seems overwhelming that we can be forced out of an old way of thinking and eventually into a new way of being in our lives.

This process of forced expansion occasions the evolution of our mind. »

We can end this chapter on trauma by studying the physiology of it.

Let us begin by a quick reminder about the fight or flight response. When a danger occurs in nature, an animal has 2 choices: Fight the danger or run away (flight) from it. A 3rd and less used option is freezing.

The Sympathetic Nervous System mobilizes the body's resources under stress and induce the fight-or-flight response. The Parasympathetic Nervous System stimulates rest and digestive activity. New understandings of the vagus nerve theorize that the dorsal branch of the vagus nerve activates the "freeze" response when other survival strategies fail (e.g. fight or flight). About this, Stephen Porges, Ph.D., Professor of Psychiatry at the University of Illinois, Chicago, and Director for that institution's Brain-Body Center, developed what he calls "Polyvagal Theory" to explain how our nervous system influences the way we react emotionally.

Over the course of our evolutionary history, we developed different coping mechanisms in the nervous system and these mechanisms are hierarchical:

1. The oldest system helps to conserve energy.
2. The next part mobilizes us.
3. The most evolved part helps to self-soothe and engage socially.

When we are the subject of a traumatizing experience, this is what chronologically happens:

1. First, we look for social cues. We use the facial muscles to self soothe - including the ears. We eat or drink, we listen to music, and we talk to people to calm down. There's a link between the nerves that regulate the face and the nerves that regulate the heart and lungs.
2. Then we go into fight and flight behaviors.
3. Then we use the very old dorsal vagal system, the freeze or shutdown mechanism, and we're out.

As we have seen earlier, when mammals are threatened, they fight, flight or freeze. If the mammal freezes but isn't killed, it has to "thaw" the freeze and it does this by shaking vigorously. This neurogenic shaking releases the mammal from the cycle of trauma by "turning off" the dorsal branch of the vagus system. The problem is that human beings have socialized ourselves out of our natural tremoring response. You can understand now why a « shaking asana » practice around Svadhisthana helps to heal a trauma.

16 YOGA AND ADDICTION

Yoga can also help with addictions. We will see here why and how. Before that, we have to define what an addiction is.

For Gabor Maté - is a retired Hungarian-born Canadian physician with a special interest in childhood development and trauma. Furthermore, in their potential lifelong impacts on physical and mental health, including addictions and a wide range of other conditions. An addiction is - « *any behavior that has negative consequences but is associated with craving and relapse, and loss of control over that behavior, despite those negative consequences. Addiction is a continuum from the highly respected workaholic at the apex of the social pyramid to the street haunted drug addict who is suffering from mental illness and facing social opprobrium at the very base. In our society, there is hardly anybody who is not affected by addiction, whether we realize it or not.* »

Risk for addiction is influenced by a combination of factors that include:
- Individual biology
- Social environment
- Age or stage of development

The more risk factors an individual has, the greater the chance that taking drugs can lead to addiction. That is why prevention is key.

A psychoactive drug can do 2 things in the brain:
- It raises the endorphins (endogenous opiates) level.
- It raises the dopamine (neurotransmitter of vitality) level.

As a point of comparison, we know that having good food raises the dopamine by 50%. Having sex raises this level by 100%. Snorting cocaine by 350%. And methamphetamine by 1200%!

The National Institute on Drug Abuse has redacted The Principles of Effective Treatment. Its 13 points are:
- Addiction is a complex but treatable disease that affects brain function and behavior.
- No single treatment is appropriate for everyone.
- Treatment needs to be readily available.
- Effective treatment attends to multiple needs of the individual, not just his or her drug abuse.
- Remaining in treatment for an adequate period of time is critical.
- Behavioral therapies—including individual, family, or group counseling—are the most commonly used forms of drug abuse treatment.
- Medications are an important element of treatment for many patients, especially when combined with counseling and other behavioral therapies.
- An individual's treatment and services plan must be assessed continually and modified as necessary to ensure that it meets his or her changing needs.
- Many drug-addicted individuals also have other mental disorders.
- Medically assisted detoxification is only the first stage of addiction treatment and by itself does little to change long-term drug abuse.
- Treatment does not need to be voluntary to be effective
- Drug use during treatment must be monitored continuously, as lapses during treatment do occur.
- Treatment programs should test patients for the presence of HIV/AIDS, hepatitis B and C, tuberculosis, and other infectious

diseases as well as provide targeted risk-reduction counseling, linking patients to treatment if necessary.

Common treatment strategies include:
- Pharmacological therapies
- 12-step programs
- Cognitive Behavioral Therapy
- Community Reinforcement Approach
- Motivational Interviewing (enhancement therapy)
- Family Systems therapy
- Contingency Management

In the West, as published by the National Institute of Health, « *Addiction is defined as a chronic, relapsing brain disease that is characterized by compulsive drug seeking and use, despite harmful consequences.* »

« *Science has taught us that stress, cues linked to the drug experience (e.g. people, places, things, moods) and exposure to drugs are the most common triggers for relapse. Medications are being developed to interfere with these triggers to help patients sustain recovery.* » NIH Pub No. 07-5605, Apr07

It is often thought that the causes of addiction are medical (genetic or brain dysfunction which can be cured by medication) or social (e.g. it is a choice).

These standard views of addiction in the West pose some issues:
- Reductionism: Tendency to reduce addiction (in terms of treatment models) to the physical, e.g. brain dysfunction or chemical imbalances.
- Disease-based: Emphasis on the negative.
- Individual issue: As opposed to a complex social problem.

It is like that because there is a cultural framework that informs us on how we understand substance use/addiction. Typically we don't analyze it because it's part of the framework of how we think. It's like a fish or a frog thinking about the water they are swimming in. As Andrew Weil, MD, says: « *Our present ways of thinking about drugs are as useless to us as a geocentric theory of the solar system. They leave us unable to describe, predict, or control the phenomena associated with drugs except in the crudest ways, as the insoluble drug problem demonstrates. Insoluble problems of this sort are always manifestations in the physical world of erroneous (that is, useless) conceptual models. » « I believe we can literally think our way out of the drug problem by changing the concepts from which it arises – the outmoded ways of thinking about consciousness in its ordinary and non-ordinary forms. »*

As Andrew Weil writes in *The Natural Mind*, straight thinking pose problems like:

- A tendency to know things through the intellect rather than through some other faculty of the mind.
- A tendency to be attached to the senses and through them to external reality.
- A tendency to pay attention to outward forms rather than to inner contents and thus to lapse into materialism.
- A tendency to perceive differences rather than similarities between phenomena.
- A tendency to negative thinking, pessimism and despair.

On the contrary, yogic worldview is holistic and synthetic. In it, causality is consciousness/spirit rather than matter and the so-called "Mind" is the cause of matter. Nowadays, coming as an evidence, quantum physics reveals the sublime reality of yoga: Everything is connected.

Also, in the yogic worldview, what exists above, exists below. The individual is thus a reflection of the society. « *Nothing arises of its own.* » - Buddha.

As said earlier, Yoga is a balance, an union, between:

- Physical: Trained by yoga poses (*asanas*), breathing practices (*pranayamas*), meditation (*dhyana*) and diet.
- Mental: Trained by ethics (*yamas* and *niyamas*), poses, meditation and service (*seva*).
- Spiritual: Trained by devotional chanting (*kirtans*), meditation and devotion (*bhakti*).

Yoga sees addiction as a spiritual malady. Its view stands on 3 main points:

- We live in a universe of desire.
- All beings desire the experience of Oneness – to "fill the God Hole".
- Every desire is a veiled desire for Oneness.

Some substance abuse is an attempt to mitigate pain. « *The quest to expand our sense of self is a core human impulse and yet, a temporary altering of boundaries only to return to a more constricted state provides limited benefits.* » - D. Simon and D. Chopra, in *Freedom from Addiction*. In Yoga, Spirit is the essence and primary causal factor.

All this parallels the Alcoholic Anonymous' point of view. As they write in their *Big Book*, sobriety is a « *daily reprieve contingent on the maintenance of our spiritual condition* » and addiction is an « *illness which only a spiritual experience will conquer* ».

Thus, the treatment, prevention and aftercare principles should derive from that which is essential - the Spirit. Our human nature (*dharma*) is only movement towards a Higher Power...

As mentioned above when quoting Dr.Gabor Maté, addiction may also be a coping mechanism for the pain of trauma.

Some yoga strategies may include:

- Mindfulness to gain perspective on pain.
- Manage and releasing pain through physical, mental, spiritual and social practices.
- Befriending the body.
- Creating safe spaces.

Flourishing – « *a state in which an individual feels positive emotion toward life and is functioning well psychologically and socially* » – should also be attained to cure an addiction.

Flourishing includes psychological flexibility and mastery of one's environment. Yet, both of these can be achieved through the diet, ethics, asanas and meditation of yoga practices.

Yoga can also help us to design a social ecology model:

A Yoga-Influenced Social Ecology Model

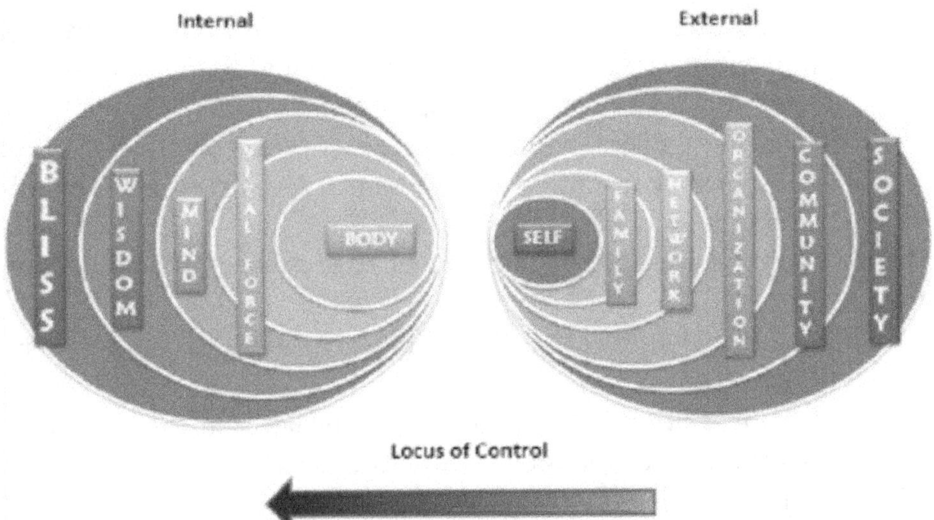

A Yoga-Influenced Social Ecology model helps to frame addiction systemically. It suggests there is not only an internal dysfunction but that there are also many factors to consider externally. Indeed, up to 70 percent of the locus of control of individual health outcomes are social (see *http://www.countyhealthrankings.org/our-approach*).

There is a real need for an integrated approach. We know that approximately only one tenth of people who would need treatment get one. The main cause (42.5%) of that is the cost of the treatment or of the insurance.
Research concludes that "broad spectrum" treatment approaches which include techniques for reducing stress and improving self-efficacy, appear to be the most useful, probably because their effects cover the widest range of factors contributing to addiction and relapse.

Yoga can help treat an addiction in a complimentary way because:
- It is holistic. Psychological and spiritual causality are as important as physical causality. Postures and breathing have proven to be an effective adjunct.

- It is oriented Towards Flourishing. Yoga balances individual flourishing or self-realization (physical, mental and spiritual) with service.
- It is accessible. It can be accessed through sport areas and other professionals and practiced at home. Many women are drawn toward body centered approaches.
- It can be applied in multiple contexts. Yoga practices can be applied in prevention, treatment, recovery, and health promotion.

The main mental and spiritual benefits of Yoga in cases of an addiction are:

- It is empowering: It is easy to learn, easy to do and cost effective.
- It helps cultivate Mindfulness: It develops impulse control, discernment in decision-making and emotional regulation, as well as interpersonal relationship skills.
- It is balancing: It develops capacity for balance and self-control, and thus reduces the need for self-medication.
- It is freeing/flourishing: It can help redirect desires and find deeper purpose and meaning in life.
- It thus helps in recovery.

Physically, Yoga:

- Improves breathing.
- Reduces cortisol.
- Decreases Blood Pressure and Heart Rate.
- Decreases Heart Rate Variability (allows the body to transition more easily between the Parasympathetic Nervous System and Sympathetic Nervous System).
- Benefits all Physiological Systems.

A global integrated Yoga approach thus acts on:

- Prevention : Practices to counter addictive tendencies/supplant cultural conditioning.
- Treatment : Practices to help sooth the nervous system and derail triggers.

- Aftercare/Reclaiming: Practices to help find renewed meaning and purpose, joy in life after treatment.
- Health Promotion: Practices which promote a healthy, Yoga oriented lifestyle. Used during all the other three phases.

It also acts at different levels:

- Spiritual: It must orient towards flourishing and has to redirect attachments from the physical towards the psychospiritual.
- Intellectual: It must challenge the mind to expand.
- Emotional: It must create internal resiliency (ability to moderate behavior in the face of adverse social effects). It also has to help cultivate Mindfulness (non-reactive calmness) and change neuro-patterning.
- Physical: Its practices must strengthen all bodily systems.
- Environmental: It must heighten subtle, aesthetic awareness.
- Social: It must create a cultural change/shift.
- Occupational: It must improve outlook and has to orient towards the positive.
- Financial: It must be cost effective.

I hope this chapter will somehow guide you to globally work with an addicted person if you have to. Of course, this has to be linked with what has been written about Svadhistana in chapter 8.

16 CONCLUSION

You now have a general overview of what the Chakras are from a scientific point of view to a more psychological/philosophical one, both based on the Yoga cosmology and Tantra, which are the real places of birth of the Chakras.

In none of the historical Hindu texts, crystals are mentioned for example. Nor are the esoteric auras. Yogis would have recognized the Koshas (the 5 Layers of Being) in them maybe...
Healing the Chakras is one of the main goal of yoga therapy (Yoga Cikitsa) and probably the best therapy for them. However, you can explore the myriads of new techniques with them and see what works for you. It also depends on what you believe in.

The most important is health, evolution and growth. I sincerely wish you the best in attaining your own goals.

THANKS

To my teachers: Deva Ram, Valérie Diaz, Yogatara L. Alessandra, Kristine « *Kaoverii* » Weber, Karen Claffey, Dr.David Frawley.

To my wife and supportive family to let me go where I want to go.

To Elaine Tobin (of Samadhi Yoga, Dublin, Ireland) and Susan Grimes for reading this book and correcting errors.

BIOGRAPHY

Stéphane Le Colas is a French yoga teacher, yoga therapist, Ayurvedic practitioner and Thai massage therapist who lives in Les Vans, in the south of France.

He discovered the Hindu philosophies thanks to his first yoga training in Nepal. Since then, he has practiced, trained and studied a lot all around the world.

Since 2013, he receives patients in his own clinic where he also gives yoga classes. He often comes to Paris to train future yoga teachers and Thai massage practitioners.
He has written 2 books about training in Ayurveda who should be translated in English in the near future.

You can get in touch with him at: stephane.lecolas@yayavara.com

www.ingramcontent.com/pod-product-compliance
Lightning Source LLC
Chambersburg PA
CBHW060755260726
48660CB00002B/630